Holly

STAND&
DELIVER

And Other Brilliant
Ways to Give Birth

Emma Mahony

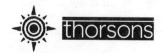
thorsons

Thorsons
An Imprint of HarperCollinsPublishers
77–85 Fulham Palace Road,
Hammersmith, London W6 8JB

The website address is:
www.thorsonselement.com

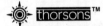

and Thorsons are trademarks of
HarperCollins*Publishers* Ltd

First published 2005

1 3 5 7 9 10 8 6 4 2

© Emma Mahony

Emma Mahony asserts the moral right to
be identified as the author of this work

Cartoons by Jonathan Pugh

A catalogue record of this book
is available from the British Library

ISBN 0 00 715399 6

Printed and bound in Great Britain by
Clays Ltd, St Ives plc

Contents

Ten Great Things About Birth **vi**
Acknowledgements **vii**
Introduction **ix**

FIRST STAGE - LET'S START AT THE VERY BEGINNING ...

Chapter 1 ... A Very Good Place to Start **3**
Chapter 2 Let's Talk about Sex, Baby **15**
Chapter 3 My Body Is a Temple **35**
Chapter 4 Free Your Mind (and Your Ass Will Follow) **55**
Chapter 5 Can You Feel It? **73**
Chapter 6 Away with the Fairies **94**

SECOND STAGE - BIRTH STORIES: BRILLIANT WAYS TO GIVE BIRTH

Chapter 7 Introduction: Water, Water Everywhere **115**
Chapter 8 Water Birth in Hospital **119**
Chapter 9 Water Birth at Home **129**
Chapter 10 Laughter Birth **136**

Chapter 11   Standing Birth **142**
Chapter 12   Induction Birth **147**
Chapter 13   Hoot Hoot Hout Birth **152**
Chapter 14   IVF Birth **158**
Chapter 15   Breech Birth **165**
Chapter 16   Twin Birth **172**
Chapter 17   Epidural Birth **183**
Chapter 18   Yoga Births **195**
Chapter 19   Caesarean Birth **203**
Chapter 20   Vaginal Birth after Caesarean
              (VBAC) **214**
Chapter 21   Helping Hands: Useful Contacts **224**

THIRD STAGE - EIGHT WEEKS TO GO

Week 32:   Where Do I Want to Give Birth? **229**
Week 33:   Antenatal Classes **235**
Week 34:   Know Your Birth Rights **238**
Week 35:   Write Your Birth Plan **242**
Week 36:   Tour the Hospital **249**
Week 37:   Glossary of Big Words Doctors Use
            around Birth **251**
Week 38:   Women Who Birth Well **257**
Week 39:   Am I in Labour? **261**
Week 40:   Physical Signs of Early Labour **263**

References **268**
Recommended Reading **271**

For my mother,
who was there from the very beginning

Ten Great Things About Birth

1 All that huffing, puffing and sweating does wonders for the skin.

2 You get your wardrobe back.

3 Everyone says how clever and wonderful you are, when the baby does most of the work.

4 At last you can join the other mothers round the table who used to stop telling their birth stories when you walked in the room.

5 You have instant rapport with every mother on the planet.

6 Without drugs, you get the most tremendous hormone high.

7 With pain-relief, you get to try different drugs legally.

8 In labour, you can act out being 'the ultimate Diva'.

9 You come the closest you'll ever get to being God, bringing forth life.

10 You get a baby to keep at the end.

Acknowledgements

A big thank-you to my favourite editor at *The Times*, Tim Teeman, for inspiration with the title, and to Johnnie Pugh for his wonderful cartoons. I must also thank those who read the manuscript when I could only look at it through gaps in my fingers – my midwives Mary Cronk MBE and Annie Francis, great mates Isabella Tree, Katy Emck, Susan Johnson and Lisa Collins, and sister-in-law Kate Houston.

Those who shared their birth stories for this book deserve special thanks for their grit and determination in getting through the editing process – harder for some than labour itself.

For their patience when the book went overdue, like all good babies, thank you to my publisher Wanda Whiteley, editor Barbara Vesey and agent Lesley Thorne.

That just leaves my family: the toddler twins Michael and Millie, who learned to charge the study door during the course of writing this, the *au pair* Judith Meissner, who tried to stop them, and my elder son Humphrey, who has shown as much interest in the birth process as my dear beloved husband, absent for all three arrivals. God bless you all.

Sorry you can't define me, sorry I break the mould,
Sorry that I speak my mind, sorry don't do what I'm told,
Sorry if I don't fake it, sorry I curse for real,
I will never hide what I really feel.

Christina Aguilera, *Stripped*, 2003

The great thing about childbirth is that it is the last time you can behave appallingly, swear, lay down the law, shriek, groan and bash your husband in the chest, and be forgiven. You are the star, the primadonna; make the most of it. Once the new star arrives, to the sound of your last furious swear-word, you will have to behave again, and be gentle and self-sacrificing. Enjoy your last fling.

Libby Purves, *How Not to Be a Perfect Mother*, 2004

Introduction

I promise not to wave joss sticks, play whale music or bombard you with photographs of women in labour and babies being born. There is no free video of 'Stephanie's Labour' on offer (which instantly put a stop to my husband attending another antenatal class). The only graphic pictures are painted in words, which, in their reading, I hope will give you a clearer picture of what you want. Cartoons from my talented *Times* colleague Jonathan Pugh also attempt to lighten a subject that you may feel is unlightenable (little do you know yet that if you could only laugh your way through labour, your birth might be trouble free).

After my first baby, I used to joke to the newly pregnant that 'birth was over-rated'. I had had a typical 'natural' birth with plenty of medical intervention – IV drip, syntocinon to strengthen contractions, foetal monitoring, epidural, stitches, syntometrine injection to deliver the placenta. I didn't understand why medics and midwives were intent on this sort of delivery as being the holy grail for women. OK, I got to leave the hospital earlier than the women who had caesareans, and I didn't have to wear the ugly white legwarmers to prevent blood clots, but I was still waddling around with the rest of the ward, feeling like I had been bucked off a rodeo bronco.

I laughed cynically at the tales of Sheila Kitzinger describing birth as a giant orgasm, and at my friends who were forgoing pain relief for a more intense experience. I had yet to understand that while my delivery was described as 'vaginal' (an adjective I loathe, so I have kept its use to the bare minimum in this book), there was little that was 'natural' or 'normal' about it. ('Normal childbirth is now the recognized medical term for birth without intervention; 'natural' is out of fashion.) I had had glimpses of what it might have been like – giggling uncontrollably with my girlfriend Lisa in the delivery room and connecting strongly with my midwife before the epidural needle was put in – but nothing that suggested an epiphany.

Well, the epiphany came at my second birth, driven not out of desire for something better but out of fear of something worse. When my doctor told me at my 30-week check-up that one of my twins was lying across my stomach, and therefore I would have to deliver them both in an operating theatre with 12 people present, I froze. And when he announced that the first could be delivered normally and the second by caesarean section, I didn't sleep properly for two weeks. My dreams were full of glinting knives and open wounds, with people watching me perform an impossible act. There must be an alternative, I thought, falling back on a journalistic habit of researching the subject over and over, calling hospitals and organisations, speaking to anyone who would listen. I knew I didn't want the huge upheaval of a major operation followed by newborn twins and a demanding toddler to care for. Where would family bonding fit into that? I felt resentful that I was being railroaded into something that I didn't want or felt I needed. And now I understand that a bad birth is not one that ends up with an emergency caesarean, but one where you feel coerced into something that you don't feel you need. My doctor's prognosis was a frightening ending to an easy pregnancy. I was deeply unhappy, and set about on a journey to get the birth I wanted – a journey which inspired me to write this book.

Knowledge and support were my two weapons in the fight to do it my way. And, having achieved it, assisted by two remarkable midwives, I now understand that a good birth is the best present a mother can give herself. The less intervention from other people, the quicker the recovery (the quicker the recovery, the better for all the family). For all my talk of 'birth being over-rated', I suddenly understood that it was under-rated. Thousands of women are being denied the opportunity to have a really good birth experience because they are unaware of the politics of pregnancy. They don't know they have rights despite current hospital protocols, shortage of midwives and cultural indifference to their plight.

Because of this indifference, the spiritual and psychological effects of being prodded and poked in hospital, or monitored like a bomb that is about to explode, have often been overlooked. The darker side of a poor birth experience may be mentioned in hushed whispers to health visitors or close friends, but new mothers are often so overwhelmed by the demands of looking after a new baby, or so grateful for its safe arrival, that they are unable to speak out for themselves at the time.

When a birth goes well, however, it is an 'uplifting', 'empowering' and 'intoxicating' experience, as all the birth stories in the second part of this book affirm. Someone who has felt in charge and in control of her birth is in a good frame of mind to bond with her baby, to nurture, nurse and wallow in those precious twilight few days that follow the beginnings of life. A good birth produces hormones, especially when breast-feeding, that shore up a woman's reserves and help her to feel confident about herself and her own judgement for days, weeks, months and years afterwards. If a mother can look back at the birth and think, 'Well, I certainly gave that my best shot,' then she can take that confidence into dealing with the scraps in the play-ground that follow.

This book argues that mother and baby are so closely entwined from the beginning of the baby's life, that anything that is good for the mother, is good for the baby, too. I don't buy a doctor's diagnosis that a pregnant woman is being 'selfish' if she wants something other than the standard hospital fare. If she's looking after herself, she's looking after her baby, too. It's not for nothing that the flight crew on board an aircraft tell parents to put on their own oxygen masks first before helping their children.

The birth stories told here are all experiences with positive outcomes. This is not so the book joins the shelves of cuddly toys and sentimental parenting magazines, where impossibly beautiful models nurture perfect babies and tell of their hospital deliveries with exclamation marks and phrases like, 'and then he just popped out!' My view is that women will be given enough warnings and negative advice throughout their pregnancy from well-meaning medical professionals and tactless strangers without hearing more from me. I am neither a medical professional nor, I hope, a tactless stranger, just someone eager to pass on the advantages of getting it right first, second, third or fourth time around.

The women interviewed have all held on to their sense of self in spite of being bossed about by the establishment. Their stories are deeply personal and many are told in detail, sometimes with milligrammes of blood loss, in the hope that they might inspire others to try for something better. Some of the women have given birth abroad, in Spain and America, countries with even higher intervention rates than Britain. I hope their positive experiences will build up your confidence, as a few good birth stories did for me when I was casting around for alternatives to my twins' birth.

There is nothing to fear from reading any of the following chapters, only something to gain. It may be the knowledge that a contraction at its most painful peak lasts only 90 seconds, or that labour might stop suddenly on arrival in hospital because of the rush of adrenalin that comes with being moved to a new and unfamiliar place. The experiences include my own, because my own fight to have my twins normally challenged most of the so-called 'birth rights' that are accepted as standard by our National Health Service. Like all the other stories included, it has a positive outcome. The birth of my twins was a turning-point for me in understanding why the opportunity to have a good birth should be every woman's right.

FIRST STAGE

LET'S START AT THE VERY BEGINNING ...

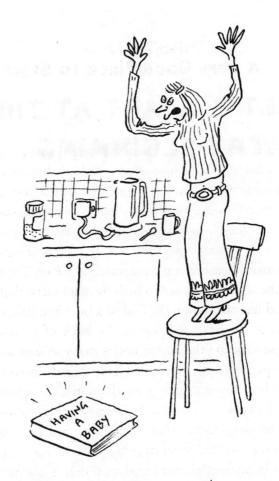

1

... A Very Good Place to Start

From the moment I realized as a little girl that my biological destiny was to have a baby, childbirth hung over my head like the sword of Damocles. Unless you are a child of a flower-power mother, and strew daisies on the floor while Mummy laboured in a yurt, birth seems a frightening and mysterious act. You know it's going to be awful because you have watched *ER* on TV, and seen the actresses pinned to beds by machinery, flailing around like salmon on the end of a line. You believe it is just as likely to happen in the back of your car, because these are the horror stories that you read about in the papers. And, most of all, you are convinced that it will hurt more than having all your teeth removed with string and a doorknob, because every stand-up comedian has cracked that joke (and no one ever heckles). Our cultural conditioning around birth is so firmly implanted on our mind map that it is amazing women fall pregnant in the first place (well, perhaps not, post-*Sex and the City*). We all live under the illusion that a 'cure' will be found during those nine months of gestation.

Well, I'm here to convince you today that birth can be fun. Say it extremely quietly, but there are plenty of women who have actually *enjoyed* giving birth. So much so, that they want to go and do it all over again AS SOON AS IT IS OVER (now you understand the hushed whispers). Don't believe all the doomsayers. Birth does not have to be like sitting O levels unprepared. If it goes right, it can be a wonderful, transforming, empowering experience that can change your image of yourself and your life for the better. I'm not saying it won't hurt. The 'ring of fire' has never been more aptly named. I'm just saying that pain and pleasure go hand in hand, especially if you add to the cocktail some powerful hormones to help it all along.

The birth of a baby is a defining moment in every woman's life, and the better it goes, the easier her transition into motherhood. So, how do we rid ourselves of all the cultural conditioning that makes us think that birth is a bad thing, a terrifying and horrible experience to be endured rather than enjoyed? Through cultural *unconditioning*.

Cultural Unconditioning

This is going to be very hard. You need to think about all those frightening little snapshots of birth that you have picked up over your non-childbearing years, write them down, screw up the paper and throw them in the bin. How you think and feel about birth is going to have a bigger effect on your eventual labour than that epidural that you have already booked. If you can look forward to it, have confidence in yourself and trust in the physiological process, then you're already halfway there.

Getting to this point is not always an easy ride. Somewhere in your psyche there is the shock of your first impression of birth. For me it was a video shown at primary school, of two legs and a human baby coming out between them. It was probably a biology class, but all I remember is looking away, shocked by the bloody violence of it all. Distanced in a clinical way by the medium of video, it became a scene from *Alien* rather than a sacred moment. Even then I could see that birth should be an intimate and private event, not open to voyeurs.

But if that image shocked me at a tender age, it did at least clear up how babies get out. Before that I believed they came out of my tummy button, an otherwise seemingly pointless part of the body.

Assumptions and ignorance about our bodies is rife among even the most educated women, and pregnancy is a good time to reacquaint yourself with your body. One 70-year-old midwife from southern Arkansas described how, when she was in labour with her first baby, she, too, didn't know where the baby was going to come out. At a conference in the 1980s she related: 'When I was alone in labour, I looked all over myself. I had a mirror and was looking all over my body. When I opened my mouth, I thought "That must be it!" When I saw that little thing in the back [her uvula], I thought that was the baby's big toe. I thought I was going to have to throw up the baby. It wasn't till the midwife came and washed between my legs that I suddenly realized where the baby was going to come out!'[1] Most of you will be further along on these issues than the midwife and my younger self, and some of you may even have studied the birth pictures in Dr Miriam Stoppard's and Sheila Kitzinger's pregnancy books. Once again, you are wiser (and braver) than I am. I still have to peep at shots of other people's births through my fingers – three babies later – and not because I get distracted by the beards and long hair in the photos (for some strange reason, all birth books only feature Seventies' casualties). If you, too, cannot stomach these images, don't worry. It won't affect your labour. When it comes to your birth, you will be heading up the important part, up top. You can leave the messy stuff to the professionals.

Doctors and the Medics

When you go into hospital – a place that will always bring up some anxiety of being ill or visiting sick relatives – you do so as an intruder. As a woman you are not ill, just pregnant, but as you sit in the waiting room as one of many, you may begin to experience new pinpricks of fear that weren't there before. In the ultrasound department, this fear may be coaxed out by giant posters on the wall showing photographs of your baby *in utero* looking like a visitor from outer space. Other posters will carry information about how you could already be harming your baby by smoking or drinking. In the waiting room there will be more posters of mothers cradling a newborn with a headline telling you Why Breast Is Best or another showing a baby sucking on a bottle of sugar, warning of the perils of giving juice in a bottle. The hospital atmosphere itself might make you start thinking new thoughts: 'Will this baby be all right?' or 'Why do they want me to take a blood and urine test? Does everyone have these, or can they see that I am a bit thinner/-fatter/taller/smaller than the woman next to me?'

Sometimes, talking to a doctor can be more confusing than enlightening, as strange words are used, as if you were already in the know: 'We are measuring the nuchal fold,' says the radiographer. 'We are looking for protein in the urine,' says the midwife, as if you had some understanding of its significance. The use of language like this builds a barrier between you and the people with the stethoscopes round their necks, and often you feel a little more helpless and a little more ignorant than before you went in.

Of course the picture I am painting may be far worse than in your corner of the country. Here in London every hospital antenatal appointment is double-booked, so you can wait over two hours for your precious five minutes with the consultant. Even in those five minutes, if you have a medical student present the doctor may not be addressing you but teaching while talking.

Testing, Testing, One, Two, Three

As well as the brief chats with the doctor, there are also all sorts of tests that you may have in your pregnancy. The main thing you need to know about all these tests is that of all the 760,000 women who fall pregnant in the UK every year, only a tiny, tiny percentage will have to alter the course of their pregnancy after being screened. Some of the tests, such as routine screening for gestational diabetes (where you are given a glucose drink to take beforehand and, unsurprisingly, your blood sugar levels go wild) are being abandoned now anyway. Peter Brocklehurst, Director of the National Perinatal Epidemiology Unit, has this to say about the GTT (Glucose Tolerance Test): 'The test is unreliable, doctors do not know how to treat it, and anxiety in the minds of the woman and her carers could be raised, increasing the risk of the pregnancy ending in a Caesarean.'[2]

I'm not suggesting that some of these tests don't have a place. The urine test to find out whether there is a certain protein in the pee to indicate pre-eclampsia (a pregnancy-induced condition that is treatable by early delivery of the baby) is a life-saver. But for the hundreds of thousands of women who are tested routinely during their pregnancies, and then retested because the result was mis-read or read as a 'false positive' – and who sometimes having to wait weeks for the result – this most magical time can turn into a fearful one. There is a lot to be said for ignorance being bliss, and my mother would argue that her 1960s generation, pre-ultrasound, was a lot better off when they simply looked forward to starting a family come what may. And this from a woman who didn't know she was carrying twins until she went into labour!

Ultraconfusing Ultrasound

While ultrasound has its uses (such as assessing more accurate dates, identifying twins and the presentation of the baby for delivery at the end of the pregnancy), it carries with it ethical dilemmas that far outweigh its uses, and any mother who doesn't want to be scanned during pregnancy is quite within her rights to refuse it.

When you learn that 20 years ago, when scanning was in its infancy, thousands of women were scared silly by being told their babies had 'golf balls' in the brain (which turned out to be perfectly healthy brain tissue), it reminds you how recent all this new technology is. The other day, a woman rang the AIMS helpline in tears when a sonographer told her to 'come back next week, I can't see the baby's head'.

Some radical groups maintain that the effects of ultrasound on growing babies and adults in later life have never fully been researched. While the effects are obviously nowhere near as dramatic as the rise in childhood leukaemia after X-rays were used on pregnant women (and Britain was the last country to stop irradiating pregnant women), it nevertheless makes you wonder why we are exposing something as fragile as the beginnings of life to unproven technology.

What is also forgotten in the rush to wave the magic radiographer's wand is how vulnerable pregnant women are to information. It's no surprise that most women don't want to know the sex of their child in this country (it is given as a rule in the States – unless the parents specifically request otherwise). We want that growing baby to be as protected as possible, a mystery up until the moment he or she is born. We don't always want early expectations heaped upon him or her because of gender, size or some minor birth defect.

My first son was born with a cleft-lip and palate that was corrected by plastic surgery when he was three and six months old, and I am still glad that the ultrasound department failed to pick up this 'anomaly'. It would have added anxiety and worry to the whole family during an otherwise stress-free pregnancy. I wouldn't have changed the course of my pregnancy knowing this, but I might have looked up unregulated sites on the internet and then worried myself stupid with other people's tales of woe.

Ultrasound is technology without responsibility. It is you, not the radiographer, who has to deal with the fall-out of whatever probability ratio the scan brings up, and whatever further tests you might be offered. As the Government announces plans to mass-screen every woman in the UK (at a cost of £153 million to us taxpayers), few people have questioned why. Some groups for people with disabilities have even described the decision as 'mass eugenics' by another name. One woman who had decided that she did not want ultrasound rang up the doctor's surgery to inform them that she did not want to have her 13-week scan. The receptionist became shirty with her about her decision, and wouldn't let her cancel. Finally, to put an end to the discussion, this woman simply reminded the receptionist that her baby was really none of the receptionist's business.

So, before you even go in for your scan, discuss the bigger picture with your partner. Talk about what you can cope with as parents, and then decide on what you'll do on that basis. Don't feel you have to be put on the conveyor belt without a choice.

Don't Worry, Be Happy

All this talk is really an attempt to shake up a few accepted views about what happens to you during your pregnancy, and to get you thinking about what you want for yourself and your new family. You have all the answers, it may just require digging a little deeper to find them.

For example, **all women know deep down where they would feel comfortable and safe giving birth**. Even if your reasons might seem ridiculous to someone else, you know best. My mother wanted to have my elder brother at home in Norfolk because she was convinced that her first-born might get switched in the hospital nursery at night. Fortunately she had a sympathetic doctor who agreed to a home birth to save her worrying further. My 11-lb brother (ouch!) was born with a fire flickering in the grate, the midwife knitting in the armchair, chucking her cigarette butts into the fire as the hours wore on (my, how times have changed). Who is to say my mother was wrong, or should have been persuaded to do otherwise (as she would have today when the scan showed a baby of that size)? Who is even to say that her worst fear might not have come true, as women are often spookily intuitive during pregnancy, and seem to know things that are not explainable in a rational way?

So, don't be downhearted by all the negativity surrounding our birth culture today, **try shocking everyone around you by announcing that you are looking forward to the birth**. You have already made a miracle by creating that baby inside of you, so why shouldn't further miracles happen – such as enjoying the big day?

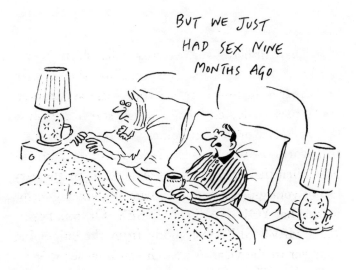

2

Let's Talk about Sex, Baby

If you have hitherto worn piecrust collar shirts, below-the-knee A-line skirts and sensible shoes, then pregnancy is the time to review your image as a woman. If you have traded on being a sexless sort of person in the workplace or in your domestic persona, a sensible, trustworthy sort who doesn't sleep around with the boss, then that *ain't gonna work no more*. By the very fact of your growing bump you are announcing to the world that YOU HAVE HAD SEX. Or, one hopes, YOU HAVE SEX. Everybody from the sniggering teenager to the vicar at church can now see this for themselves. That hitherto most private and mysterious part of yourself is paraded on view, saying 'Look everybody, I am a fertile woman who is sexy enough for someone to want to impregnate me!' You may think that your pregnancy dungarees and Doc Marten boots are saying something else, but this is the message on the most basic level that the world is receiving.

This is no small matter. I can still remember realizing in a Biology class that I was a result of my parents 'doing it'. I was appalled. I could only compute the idea by believing that they had done it just the two times in the marriage to produce us children. From then on, in my pre-teen state, pregnant women on the street were not gorgeous goddesses but women who had done that unspeakable act – yuk! Put that thought into the mind of teenage boys and you can see why 'denial' is not the place you should be right now.

Sex and Birth

Although you may never learn this at your hospital appointments, confronted by doctors with stethoscopes around their necks, sex and birth are closely linked. A good healthy approach to sex can help produce a good, healthy birth outcome. That doesn't mean to say that if you can't face a session in the sack until after the birth that you may as well book in for a C-section. There are many ways to fry a fish (sorry), and in the hand-out that accompanies the pregnancy Pink Kit from New Zealand (visit www.commonknowledgetrust.com for a look), there is a line that says 'Women who birth well touch themselves appropriately to facilitate the experi-ence.' If that line makes you go 'eek' (and not because of the mangled syntax) then you need to dig a little deeper and ask yourself why. Being into your body and finding yourself beautiful in your pregnant state may require a thought-makeover (more cultural uncondi-tioning). After all, waif-like models are the ideal, aren't they? Well, no, actually. Try asking any red-blooded male, and don't be surprised by his answer. Some men find pregnant women very sexy, and if you happen to show your bump in Greece you will be accosted by Greek men keen to rub your tummy for good luck. Just remember that the *Sun* does not sell 2 million copies every day because of its acute political sensibilities.

In the deeply unsexy environment of a hospital, however, where death and disease reign, it is not surprising that sex is the furthest thing from all of our minds. If it is discussed at our antenatal classes, it is discussed in a clinical sort of way with off-putting words like 'penetration', 'intercourse' or 'stimulation' used. Now, if George Clooney were to show up and take the class over a glass of wine in a bar, things might be different. But near the Sanitary Waste bucket next to the foetal monitor, lovemaking is never going to be at the forefront of anyone's mind.

So, before I pull the rabbit out of the hat and reveal how sex and birth are so closely linked, I need to break the postnatal conspiracy of silence over the issue of sex *after* birth, to show you why it is worth doing a little extra work on yourself and your relationship in your pregnant state. If you are in a relationship, ignoring the importance of sex is never going to work. After money, it is the main reason why couples fight. It will raise its head (as it were) at some stage after the birth, and you have a lot more time and energy to explore your feelings before the baby comes than afterwards. Sex is also going to become an issue after the birth anyway, when you suddenly find yourself in a twilight world where breastfeeding, exhaustion, resentment, broken nights and a grumpy partner make the good old days of a Sunday morning romp the stuff of fantasy. Now, not later, is the time to wise up to your womanhood, even if you would really rather prefer to flick through cute baby catalogues.

Sorting Out Your Sex Life

Many women won't need any prompting to look at their sexual selves, and those lucky types will find that the pregnancy hormones will make them feel gorgeous, glowing, blossoming and at the very height of their sexual prowess. Already up the duff, so no thought of contraception necessary, they can toss their inhibitions to the wind, revel in their burgeoning breast size and feel confident in expecting a little bit more gratification from their partners in return for bestowing their bounty upon them. Even these women, vital and brimming with life, will need to protect themselves from other females, some of whom will be unable to stop themselves from cutting them down in their prime. If you do receive a bitchy comment about your increasing size, remember to quip back how much your partner *just loves the new you.* Then practise your Miss Piggy hair flick and walk away.

Whatever Floats Your Boat

There is no easy way to bring up the topic of bisexuality, so I am going to launch right in there. First, it often appears in fantasy form during pregnancy. It may be hormones, or something to do with your changing shape and your body image changing with it, or it may be the increasingly unwelcome notion of a rough, masculine touch when all is taut and tender. In *Becoming a Mother* by Kate Mosse (no, not the supermodel, wake up at the back, please) one woman explains rather explicitly:

I used to think 'I wish I was with a woman.' I had this feeling all the way through my pregnancy and this was for two reasons: one, all my women acquaintances, friends, were so appreciative of my changing shape. I had so many compliments about my bump, I can't tell you, and they genuinely meant it, they think it's beautiful. And two, because I just thought a woman would know how to make love in such a way (what I wanted was to be licked, sucked; even being touched with fingers could be too intrusive and painful) ...

So much for the fantasy, but what of the reality? Well, out of bi-curiosity I asked eight of my closest friends if they had ever snogged a girl or more, and a (surprising) six said 'yes'. Their forays usually took place in their early twenties (and usually under the influence of drink or drugs, where boundaries are fudged anyway) but that straw-poll indicates quite how on your doorstep the bisexual issue might be. Of those bi-curious six, five have gone on to get married and have children, so their experiences mostly point to a flowering of their early sexual selves. One even suggested that 'all women are fundamentally gay', but that we have switched off that part and chosen not to pursue it. While I wouldn't necessarily agree, I would say that bisexuality is still taboo in a way that lesbianism no longer is. A lesbian who has 'come out' has weathered the reactions and disapproval of family, friends and neighbours to be her own person and find support within a recognized group. Someone who has had bisexual dalliances might be nothing more than keen to cover it all up.

Pressing my confessing friends further, I find that their flirtations with the same sex can be put down to everything from horniness to boarding school and missing Mummy, from a painful break-up to becoming a radical feminist, from confusion to vulnerability – all understandable emotions and situations that didn't determine their future sexual proclivities. But carrying around the knowledge of these forays has been a weight for some of them.

If you sit in one of the six seats occupied by my friends, now might be a good time to process this aspect of yourself. Write it out in your pregnancy journal, speak your mind to a friend who's also been there, or raise the subject generally with your partner (even the most prudish man entertains top-shelf magazine fantasies of

Dos Lesbianos en la Piscina). Don't just stamp it down, and don't believe that because you are now entering a new, ordered, conservative world of pinnies and nappies that you can suppress this side of yourself. You can't. It will come back and haunt you, and may translate in the most unexpected way. One of the six admitted that the ten-year-old memory had stopped her from pursuing friendships with other local mothers, in case there might be something 'inappropriate' in her manner. The only thing inappropriate in this loyal friend's behaviour was her own self-sabotage because of her 'guilty secret'. Don't let that be you.

If, like me, you reside in the other two-eighths of the group, a hetero square-o that has never crossed that line, don't be quick to judge anyone else. Otherwise, you might find yourself looking back from the other side of forty, putting out the milk bottles after tucking up the children in bed, thinking 'Mmm, maybe in my pursuit of men of all sizes, ages, shapes and colours, I missed out on something here.' Perhaps 'love is universal' (as one friend offered by way of explanation for her own Sapphic sorties). But you, for all your suburban riches, will never know. And Madonna, Britney and Christina are never likely to ask you to join them on stage to find out.

Sex to Start Labour

A week overdue with my first child, I arrived in hospital barely in labour and announced that I wasn't leaving until I had had the baby. I was fed up with being pregnant and felt like a lumbering elephant. After my contractions had slowed to nothing again, a midwife walked into the room and whispered to me that I should go home and make love to my husband 'because sperm can start labour'. Certainly nobody had told me at the antenatal classes that semen is the richest source of prostaglandin, a hormone that acts as a trigger to start labour. I wish they had. I could have done with a bit of fun at that stage, and it may have saved me a few hot curries and bumpy car rides up the road. Especially when the gels and pessaries that I was then offered to get things going were 'synthetic prostaglandin' – in other words, artificial spunk.

Reading through my pregnancy diary for this chapter, I was surprised to find that my very last entry while I was overdue and waiting to go into labour involved a long and detailed sexual fantasy that I had at 4 a.m. in the morning. Trying to decipher my scrawly handwriting in the dark was less interesting than the retrospective realization that on some level perhaps my mind and body were trying to work together to get labour going. To think that if I had told my sleeping husband that fantasy in the morning, I might have got labour off to a quicker start. As it was, the last sentence

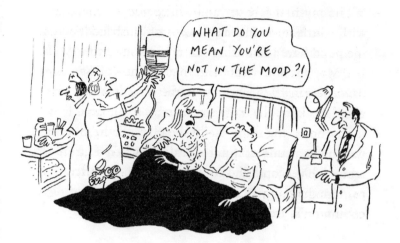

of my pregnancy journal reads 'Outrageous!' Outrageous? That was nothing compared to what was about to follow.

Listen to the Hippies, Man

While my first labour might have got going quicker with a little more intimacy, some of our friends across the pond have been using sex in birth since the 1960s. Ina May Gaskin wrote the first edition of *Spiritual Midwifery* in 1975, and says in the Introduction, 'Generally speaking, the more comfortable a woman is living in her body, the more easily she gives birth.' She was writing at a time of hippie idealism, when a group of around 300 people had come together in San Francisco to tour the country in camper vans until founding a commune in rural Tennessee called The Farm.

Ina May, after attending the births of women on the road trip, went on to qualify as a midwife and keep records that prove that intense emotional support and trust in the physiological process produce great birth outcomes. There were 11 births on the road before they settled in Tennessee, and today, after 2,028 pregnancies, 95 per cent completed at home and only a 1.4 per cent Caesarean rate (compare that with 30 per cent in some British hospitals), The Farm's statistics must beat any other birth centre in the world. Here are a few of the more experimental lessons they learned on the way.

A Kiss on the Lips May Be ...

... all that you need to get you through labour. Believe it or not, there is an extraordinary correlation between a relaxed mouth and a ripe cervix. Not that extraordinary when you consider that a good kissing session probably preceded your current state of falling pregnant in the first place. Ina May Gaskin encouraged the women she attended to practise 'horse lips', or blowing raspberries, after discovering a direct link between a relaxed mouth and lips and, well, the *labia*, or other set of lips we girls have. During one birth on The Farm, a four-year-old girl stood beside her labouring mother demonstrating how to blow better raspberries between contractions. The mother copied her, laughing, and shortly afterwards a new sibling arrived.

Also effective on the lip front is French kissing your partner (now imagine how *that* would go down with the starchy midwives on an NHS labour ward). In *Spiritual Midwifery*, a Farm resident called Marilyn, who had already had two children, describes her home birth:

Rather quickly, those monumental tidal waves of energy which women on The Farm called 'rushes' [contractions] came upon me for the third time. Had I discussed this with Gerald beforehand? I don't remember. He was reclining next to me, and at the start of a heavy contraction, I found his mouth and we French kissed. Whew! Here comes another! We kissed again, from the start to the finish of the contraction. My mouth must have been opened cavernously wide, because later Gerald told me I nearly sucked the denture out of his teeth. I'm glad he chose to tell me this later. I didn't need anything inhibiting me while I was testing the midwives' adage: 'It's that loving, sexy vibe that puts the baby in there in the first place, and the same loving, sexy vibe will get the baby out.' And it did. I didn't tear with Annie, who weighed six pounds.

The lips manoeuvre is not something you even need to wait until the birth to try. If you have been with your partner for so long that you often forget to include kissing in your lovemaking any more, try out Marilyn's denture-sucking French kiss with a view to what's happening down below at the same time.

Tits Oot for the Lads

That loving sexy vibe is not only confined to the mouth. If I told you that in hospital you are often hooked up to an IV drip (which is almost routine procedure in some places) and then given synthetic oxytocin to get your labour started, you wouldn't be in the least bit surprised. If you now learn that real oxytocin is produced naturally by your body as you start to make love, and is that warm feeling that rushes through you during a heated embrace, then you might be a little more shocked.

As our own resident High Priestess of Natural Birth, Sheila Kitzinger describes in *Birth Your Way*:

For many women the very gentle arousal produced by nipple stimulation, carried out by you or someone else, may produce contractions if continued for 20 minutes or so at a time. Stroke the nipples with your fingers, rolling, sucking or licking them [tricky unless you are a dog], or rest a warm face cloth on your breasts, lifting it off when it cools, dipping it in hot water, and pressing it against the nipples again.

Sheila also notes that 'Masturbation will also produce contractions and, because it is possible to have an orgasm very quickly and to experience multiple orgasm with self-stimulation, it may be a more effective method than intercourse in starting off labour.' Orgasm in a woman produces waves of contractions in the clitoris, vagina and uterus, and opens the cervix. Ho, ho, ho. Even if it doesn't work, you can at least have fun trying.

Try Some New Positions

Good positions to make love in and good positions to birth the baby also have some things in common. For example, **the best way for most women to give birth is on their hands and knees, doggy style**. Now it is difficult to adopt this position without immediately being transported back to some dubious session with the lights out. Mid-labour with my first baby, when the midwife came in to find me on my hands and knees being massaged by my birth buddy Lisa, I felt she'd opened the door on some porno movie. 'I think she thinks we're some sort of lesbian double act,' I whispered, grabbing the gas and air back off my so-called friend who was sucking away on it. The disapproving midwife left the room, and we both fell about laughing.

For the lazy among you, unwilling to try new positions and therefore get yourself in the mood to try any position that feels comfortable on the big day, may I offer you the wise words of the obstetrician Professor Roberto Caldeyro Barcia: 'The only position worse than lying on your back for birth is hanging by your heels from a chandelier.'[1] And there's another one for you to try.

I'll Have What She's Having

While no one can promise you an orgasmic birth in your new negligée, there are plenty of people who do have one. Ina May Gaskin asked 151 women who had birthed on The Farm in Tennessee if any had experienced orgasm at birth, and a staggering 21 per cent said yes! If your first reaction is that they are lying, why would they bother? Marilyn of denture-sucking fame was fairly typical:

My last birth was very orgasmic in a sustained sort of way, like I was riding on waves of orgasmic bliss. I knew more what to expect, was less afraid, and tried to meet and flow with the energy rather than avoid or resist as I had first time. The effect was probably mostly psychological in that it gave me tremendous satisfaction just to have accomplished such a difficult passage safely. I felt great for months afterwards, which helped me to feel positive about myself in general. This in turn affected how I felt about myself sexually. I also think that, for me, learning to let go and let my body take over in labour helped me to tap into a part of me that I never knew before, and helped me to feel more willing to let go while making love.

Many women find that after giving birth, a few weeks or months down the line, sex becomes better and better with their partner, and some experience orgasm for the first time. Might this be you?

Sorry Darling, I've Got a Headache

What if you just don't feel like doing it? Pregnancy may drip-feed you hormones that soften and engorge your yoni, make the clitoris more sensitive, and hit a triple jackpot with making the lubricating cervical glands work overtime, but what use is that if you are forever rushing to the loo to chuck up your Boots sandwich? It is all very well wandering around in a state of semi-arousal, but if this is accompanied by tiredness and aching breasts, then what's the point? My favourite line in Vicki Iovine's *Best Friend's Guide to Pregnancy* is when she describes the urge to hit her husband over the head with a bedside lamp when he goes near her breasts in the first three months. Not everyone is in the mood at the beginning.

Although Dr Miriam Stoppard in the *New Pregnancy and Birth Book* says, 'The majority of women I have spoken to about sex and pregnancy have almost universally felt that sex was better than ever,' I reckon she conducted most of her research in the nymphomaniac district of Amsterdam. The truth is that sex is a very complicated issue among individuals, let alone couples, and it tends to be where we dump all our private and collective neuroses.

Most commonly, our body image determines how we feel as a woman. Sad to say in our post-feminist age, but if pregnancy makes you feel fat instead of gorgeous, then that is going to translate immediately into your lovemaking. The light will go firmly off when undressing, some of you may reach for the chocolate box rather than the fruit bowl, and you just won't feel desirable. You may even subconsciously push your man away.

However, always remember that the reality is that **most men find the extra curves and roundedness of women in the early and middle flushes of pregnancy a real turn-on**. So don't you dare confuse your own feelings with those of your partner. Men are conditioned by nature to fancy fertile women, and you are a walking example of voluptuousness.

Pregnancy is the time to buy some postcards of Rubens' paintings to stick on the fridge, with white fleshy mamas breastfeeding cherubs and muscly men hovering in attendance. It'll remind you that heroin chic wasn't always fashionable.

Not Tonight, Josephine

Men do sometimes go off the idea of sex at the very end of pregnancy, however, usually when we women have finally reconciled ourselves to our fulsomeness and are suddenly prepared to test the theory of carpet burns. They also harbour fears of harming the baby in some way during a bonk, as if their huge member will puncture the amniotic sac like some Roman spear (just how big do they really think they are?). You may want to let them know as early as possible that this has never yet happened in the history of humanity. If you need to get technical, explain how a baby is protected by the amniotic sac and the walls of the uterus, and that the sperm cannot get through the mucus plug. Only if the mucus plug has come away at the start of labour should you need to refrain from making love.

Some men (and fewer women) can also find the presence of the baby off-putting in some way, as if there are three of you in on the act. This is another fear that should be winkled out and explored as early as possible, **because that presence ain't gonna go away for a while**, and will be making itself known much more vocally down the baby monitor than it is now. This might be the moment to book a dirty weekend away in some bed and breakfast in Brighton. Having nothing better to do than eat, sleep and make love should flush out this fear in full.

Above all, you can no longer take your sex life for granted in your pregnant state. If you as a woman decide to take charge of the bedroom in pregnancy, and love your body in order to give birth the best shot, there is plenty of work to be done. As all the heightened hormone level shows, your body is willing if your mind will follow. Forget feeling guilty about missing the yoga class, and substitute it for a candlelit dinner for two instead. Swop the phrase 'pelvic floor exercises' for 'romp on the floor', and put a smile back on your face. Sex got you into this mess, and sex can help get you out. So what are you waiting for? Let's go shopping.

What to Buy to Feel Sexier in Pregnancy

One friend bought pregnancy massage oil, ostensibly to massage the area under her bump that became sore at the end of a working day (the hormone relaxin softens the muscles and can sometimes cause a bit of grating around the pelvis). Asking her husband to do it as an evening ritual, she found one thing used to lead to another. (For pregnancy massage oil visit www.active-birthcentre.com.)

Another bought a good push-up bra to accentuate that great pregnancy asset – big boobs. Even if you have always been a firmly buttoned-up sort of girl, try leaving one more shirt button undone around the house, à la Sophie Dahl, during these nine months just to experiment with your new curviness. At the very least it will get you in training for breastfeeding.

Allegra tried perineal massage during pregnancy, done with her partner, using olive oil. (The perineal area is between your bum hole and your vagina.) Not a very British thing to do, but she admits: 'We just ended up laughing, it was so funny, I would kind of lie on the bed and he'd watch TV over my shoulder. That was towards the end, during the last month.' (For perineal massage oil visit www.activebirthcentre.com.)

Pregnancy tights are difficult to find and uncomfortable at the worst of times, so buy some stockings or lacy hold-ups instead. Emma did this during pregnancy and used to flash her husband as they walked out of the door in the evening, and then enjoy his extra attentiveness in the cab and during dinner. All men live in hope.

Rosie suggests buying one really sexy evening dress for the pregnancy. She invested in a designer dress, and found the designer adored doing something different for her shape. The final outfit was a skin-tight satin under-dress with a cutaway claret velvet dress coat over the top with extra emphasis in the cutting on the cleavage. Says Rosie: 'It made me feel so sexy, and everyone said they wanted to be pregnant to wear the dress.'

Exchange your dad's-old-shirt-as-a-nightie for a grown-up satiny or, if someone else is buying, silk negligée. While your gamine legs might have looked great from under the shirt before pregnancy, winceyette won't work if the legs become tree trunks. The negligée may only need to make an appearance when you are feeling in the mood, but just wearing it usually produces a male Pavlovian reaction.

Lying in bed in New York, pregnant and waiting for her husband to come home, Lois found that surfing the channels for the soft porn became a useful evening ritual. 'The sight of all these nubile young men parading around in my bedroom always seemed to get me in the mood,' she admits.

3

My Body Is a Temple

Elizabeth Gilmore set up an $800,000 birth centre in New Mexico, had the midwives employ the doctors, and brought the C-section rate down from 35 per cent to 4 per cent in the town of Taos. It has the highest out-of-hospital birth rate in the United States. I visited Elizabeth out there, interested to hear some of her Wild West views on birthing better. Here's what she said:

Have you ever seen an auction of expensive Arabian mares? I happened to catch one on the news the other day. They are raised in beautiful stalls, lovely fields full of grass, woken up every morning with hot mash. They get massaged and washed and played with, and swim in these special tanks. Because these mares are worth hundreds of thousands of dollars, and a foal up to a million dollars, they get pampered and spoiled, with ribbons woven into their hair. What if we thought that each pregnant woman was worth a million dollars, and we treated her like a princess, like an Arabian mare, and that her baby was worth millions of dollars because that baby was going to be a contributor to society?

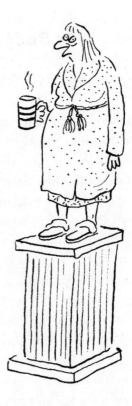
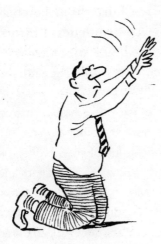

Just imagine. Because no one else is going to do it for you. Pregnancy is your time to pamper and spoil yourself.

If you are a working mother looking after a small child at home, or a working mother commuting to and from an office, then there is even more cause for some Arabian-mare treatment. If it helps to think that you are doing this for the good of your baby, rather than yourself, then so be it. Whatever it takes to keep you looking after yourself. Any of the therapies you choose to have will help you during the birth, but in ways that you probably can't see from where you are sitting now. It may be that they give you time to focus on your body, or teach you how to relax, or remind you how well you can cope with a little pain and discomfort – like my recent reflexology session taught me when I went in with blocked sinuses.

Eat Well and Multiply

Because indulging in good food is one of the few vices left to women once pregnant, I am including it as a therapy. I am not going to patronize you with lectures about the benefits of healthy eating, you know the rules. Just don't do as I did in my first pregnancy and use the lady-with-a-baby excuse to binge for nine months on chocolate and snacks. I put on two stone and produced an 8-lb baby. Second-time around, when

I binged on fruit, vegetables and anything healthy from the deli, I put on no extra weight and produced two babies weighing a total of 13lb. That's more like it.

Maternal nutrition is going to matter in the run-up to the birth (and in recovering afterwards), so do think carefully about what passes your lips. Imagine you are training to run a marathon and eat accordingly. You want to be as fit as possible for labour and new motherhood. In the first couple of months of your pregnancy you want to eat 'nutrient-dense' food because the placenta, a national-grid-like infrastructure supplying the baby, is developing.

Placenta Matters

The placenta is like a giant root system, tapping into the mother's bloodstream. As the embryo implants within the uterine wall lining, cells branch out to destroy the wall separating the mother and child and expand the diameter of the blood vessels. The mother is able neither to constrict the vessels supplying the embryo, nor to regulate the flow of nutrients to the placenta without starving herself, so the baby gains considerable control over its own intake.[1]

By the 8th week of pregnancy, the placenta composes 85 per cent of the total package and, end to end, the villi (the finger-like projections to increase the absorptive surface of the placenta) stretch about 30 miles. Once the placenta has secured the supply lines, then and only then does the baby start growing. **If you worry that morning sickness is ridding your body of all your best efforts to eat healthily, don't. There are studies to suggest that vomiting may even stimulate early placental growth.**

The most important addition to make to your healthy eating in the early days is to **eat fresh fruit and veg**. There is no need to limit your intake, eat as much as you can as often as you can. There is new research to suggest that such a diet high in vitamin C will also combat free-radical damage to blood vessels, lower blood pressure and reduce the incidence of pre-eclampsia – a dangerous condition that occurs usually in late pregnancy and requires the baby to be delivered immediately.

Also, recent research from Denmark reported in the *British Medical Journal* showed that women who **eat a diet rich in fish** during pregnancy are four times less likely to give birth prematurely. Among 8,700 women surveyed, 7.1 per cent who never ate fish had a premature delivery, yet only 1.9 per cent per cent of fish-eaters did. So, if you are still working, have smoked salmon sandwiches, along with some apples and oranges at your desk, and ignore the office vending machine.

Like most marathon runners, you will need to **drink plenty of water** (up to 2 litres a day). If you can't face water, try caffeine-free teas chilled in the fridge or the (fairly foul) raspberry-leaf tea, a good uterine-toner, found in health food shops. My American birth partner was so obsessed with my raspberry-leaf tea intake (not to be confused with a delicious Raspberry Zinger from the Twinings Exotic selection) that she was forever brewing up another cup of the tasteless soup for me as the birth approached. It is difficult to see what such a herbal remedy can achieve other than rehydrating you, but raspberry-leaf tea is strong enough to carry a warning that it shouldn't be taken before 28 weeks or by women with a history of pre-term labour. Suzannah Olivier, author of *Eating for a Perfect Pregnancy*, recommends doubling your intake as labour starts, to help things go smoothly.[2]

Suzannah Olivier is also unequivocal about the need to **take supplements**. Don't skimp and take herbal alternatives to the ones on sale in most chemists, buy the standard Pregnacare, sit it on your bedside table and make it part of your morning ritual throughout pregnancy. The same goes for folic acid during those first three months.

If, however, you are reading this on your way to the delivery suite and haven't let anything but a good healthy diet pass your lips, don't panic. Some midwives, such as Mary Cronk, believe that that is all a woman needs during her pregnancy, and that taking unnecessary supplements benefits only the manufacturers. Says Cronk: 'Supplements, particularly iron in a woman who has plenty, can imbalance the system and lead to lack of absorption of trace elements. Women eating well are usually getting all the goodies their body and baby need.'

Thinking Outside the Box of Fruit

Suzannah Olivier recommends including a few foods that might be new to your diet during pregnancy:

I recommend tree nuts, such as almonds and walnuts, seeds, pulses, pumpkin seeds, pine nuts and sunflower seeds, as well as oily fish – such as mackerel and tuna – which are particularly good nutritionally, as is lean red meat which is a source of iron and zinc, a mineral found in all protein-rich food.

Zinc and essential fats are particularly important for growth in the third trimester when the baby is putting on weight, because, if there's not enough, the baby will take it from the mother's reserves. There is one school of thought that believes that some postnatal depression may be linked to a depletion of zinc and essential fatty acids in a mother after the birth.

Make sure you add some calcium-rich food – not only milk, and yoghurt (which is predigested by bacteria so a particularly good source) but also green leafy veg, such as spinach and cabbage that contains magnesium as well.

Finally, for snacks, carry raisins and dried apricots around, because they are good sources of calcium, magnesium, potassium and iron – all needed for yours and the baby's bone health. For slow-releasing carbohydrates, oat cakes and rye crackers (particularly with mashed banana on top) will fill you up.[3]

If all the above makes you want to reach for the Dairylea, don't worry. Eat what your body wants to eat. It probably knows best.

Yoga, Walking and Swimming

The safest forms of 'aerobic' exercise to take when pregnant are walking (an hour a day is ideal), swimming (which supports all the muscles, increases blood flow and urine output, and reduces swelling) and yoga. Yoga classes are particularly good, especially if you can find or persuade a yoga teacher to set up an antenatal one, because then there is group support as well. Yoga works so well in pregnancy because it makes the most of the natural increase in suppleness due to the hormone relaxin coursing through your body. In addition, Janet Balaskas, who runs the antenatal yoga programme at the Active Birth Centre in north London, lists its benefits as: helping you to 'make friends' with your pain and to go beyond your normal limits while stretching; improving blood circulation and breathing; regulating blood pressure and heart rate; and correcting posture to help prevent backache. 'I would say that after a whole 25 years of being a childbirth educator, I've never found anything to be more potentially effective than yoga in pregnancy,' she says. Although Balaskas does not keep ongoing records of the births of her students, one year she estimated that 80 per cent of her students went on to have a natural birth without intervention – not even an epidural. 'Natural Active birth is not just for lentil eaters and brown sandal wearers,' says Balaskas, 'it is practical and safe.'

If there are no antenatal yoga teachers in your area, you can always start to do it yourself by buying one of Balaskas' books, such as *Preparing for Birth with Yoga* (Thorsons, 2003).

Scents and Sensibility

Aromatic essential oils are a great healer for those common discomforts in the last stages of pregnancy, and are particularly good for massage during labour. Take some advice, however, because certain oils should be avoided, and essential oils should not be used at all until after the first three months.

My midwife massaged me on my lower back during labour with some rose oil that she had brought back from Turkey, and it was something pleasant to do while lying in the bath before my waters broke.

Aromatherapists describe rose oil as a uterine relaxant, which helps soften the ligaments and help the pelvic bones expand, as well as being a natural antiseptic and having slight analgesic properties.

Sceptics of the benefits of aromatherapy in labour may be interested by the results of the largest clinical aromatherapy trial in Europe, which took place in the John Radcliffe Hospital in Oxford. Over a period of nine years, 8,000 mothers were offered aromatherapy in labour. Those that took it up were proved to have shorter labours with fewer drugs were used for pain-relief. There were no side-effects on the babies.[4]

One mother I met recently at the Active Birth Centre in north London was Natalie, who had no pain-relief during the birth of her breech baby, delivered standing up at home. All she had was a few drops of clary sage (another uterine tonic that is good for labour pains) put on a wet sponge and inhaled. She claims, 'It acted like gas and air, and I was practically chewing the sponge by the end!' She gave birth to an 8-lb little boy, without anyone touching her or the baby throughout the whole experience ('If anyone came near me, I just said "don't touch me!"') while two ambulances and a host of midwives waited outside the door.

The typical gripes during the last stages of pregnancy – swelling, indigestion, muscle ache and poor sleep – can all be improved with a good oily rub in the last few weeks, particularly if you can find a professional to do it for you. Stick to lavender and citrus oils for facial and body massage because there are many oils to avoid altogether.

The best carrier oil for essential oils when pregnant is sweet almond, a medium-to-light oil which protects and nourishes the skin, and is relatively pure because it is cold-pressed. While pregnant, the usual dosage of 1 drop of essential oil per 5ml of carrier oil, for facial massage, should be further diluted to 1 drop per 10ml.

Essential oil-wise, lavender is an analgesic, making it good for aches and pains, as well as relaxing (add 3 drops to a warm bath in the evening to help you sleep).

Mandarin oil is an uplifting oil and has carminative and digestive properties which help heartburn and indigestion, as well as stimulating the lymph glands – good for oedema (water-retention) and swollen ankles.

Grapefruit oil also has an uplifting effect and is good for general fatigue, circulation, and muscle stiffness.

Try sweet orange (*Citrus sinensis*) for its digestive properties, black pepper (*Piper nigrum*) as a muscular tonic, and ylang ylang (*Cananga odorata*) for calming and soothing. Denise Tiran, author of *Natural Remedies* (Quadrille, 2001) recommends that you don't use the same oil for more than three weeks, particularly in your bath water, so chop and change as you deem fit.

For labour, blend your favourites with 3 drops per 20 ml of carrier oil, and don't forget to add good old clary sage. If it worked for Natalie, it could work for you.[5]

If you can afford to go the whole hog, to find out where your nearest accredited aromatherapist is contact the International Federation of Aromatherapists at 182 Chiswick High Road, London W4 1PP (tel. 0208 742 2605) or visit their website at www.ifaroma.org. A ready-made organic labour massage oil containing lavender, clary sage and geranium can be bought from www.activebirthcentre.com, where the organic perineal massage oil is also sold.

Feet Need Love, Too

You probably already know a little about *reflexology*, where areas of the foot that correspond to the internal organs and the skeleton of your body are massaged. By massaging certain points, a trained reflexologist can tell where there are imbalances in the system. When I had bad sinusitis and a cold, the trained reflexologist Vivian Knowland massaged my toes (which relate to the sinus areas) and I ouched and eeed my way on the bed, amazed by the power concentrated in her thumbs.

Reflexology can be used to prime labour. It doesn't always work as a form of induction, but Viv chatted amiably to me about a client who had come to see her when 10 days overdue with her second baby. 'Poor woman was in a terrible state,' she said, 'The hospital had told her that she had to come in and be induced, and she really didn't want to.' So what happened, I asked, hoping that she wasn't suffering from sinus problems at the time. 'I spent some time working on her feet and she left feeling very calm. She rang me from home 10 hours later to say that she was cuddling her new baby.' Labour had apparently started as soon as she got home, followed by an easy two-hour birth in the hospital. The miracle of me-time.

Once already in labour, there are many techniques that can be used, as Suzanne Enzer details in her book *Reflexology as a Tool for Midwives*. Enzer, who has travelled as far as Australia to teach midwives and maternity reflexologists, says 'Reflexology is a superb therapy to support the natural event of childbearing and childbirth. If you have had reflexology during your pregnancy you will be in the best possible state to go through birthing. It is never too late, and if you have not had reflexology during pregnancy, it is still a wonderful complementary therapy to support birthing.' In labour, you may want to get someone to tap into some reflexology techniques and do some ankle rotations to relax the pelvis. To do this, get them to practise on someone else by asking them to hold the ankle with one hand and rotate the foot with the other hand, turning it clockwise several times and anticlockwise the same number of times. Take care to rotate the ball of the foot rather than the toes to stimulate the whole reproductive area and encourage the pelvis to relax, and include lots of gentle foot-stroking.

To find a local reflexologist, contact the Association of Reflexologists at 27 Old Gloucester Street, London WC1N 3XX (tel. 0870 567 3320) or visit www.aor.org.uk., and click on Find A Reflexologist.

Acupuncture and Shiatsu Massage

Acupuncture deserves special recognition in pregnancy because it is used with a specific technique called moxibustion, which involves the use of compressed herb sticks as heat sources above acupuncture points on the feet to turn a breech baby to head-first. What is more, it claims a 60 per cent success rate.[6] Acupuncture can also be used for other common pregnancy complaints. If you have never had it before, pregnancy is a good time to start, and it is rather an exciting treatment to have. The sensation of a fine needle being inserted into your skin and the subsequent tingling sensation, which feels like liquid evaporating on your skin as the blockage becomes unblocked, is an extraordinary feeling. In China, acupuncturists are even used to alleviate pain during labour (a sort of needle-happy TENS machine), and for anaesthesia with Caesarean sections.

Shiatsu massage, which is Japanese for 'finger pressure', has the added advantage that you don't need to take your clothes off to have it. No small bonus if, like me, you were waddling in on a cold December day. Shiatsu uses simple pressure and holding techniques and is based on Traditional Chinese Medicine, using the principles of meridians and energy lines throughout the body, like acupuncture. It increases circulation, gets rid of toxins and is a gentle way to spend an hour on the floor. I used to book my next session in a dream-like state immediately afterwards – and probably spent the best part of the twins' annual babygro budget like this.

For details of qualified therapists contact the British Acupuncture Council, 63 Jeddoe Road, London W12 9HQ (tel. 0208 735 0400) or visit www.acupuncture. org.uk and click on Find an Acupuncturist. For The Shiatsu Society, it's Eastlands Court, St Peters Road, Rugby CV21 3QP (tel. 0845 1304560) or visit www.shiatsu.org.

Birth Balls

OK, OK, you don't mind signing up for the reflexology and massage session, but you just can't face the swimming pool or even the yoga class in your current state.

Enter the Birth Ball, the final resort for those for whom exercise is a dirty word. It exercises you while you sit on it, without you having to do anything. No, it's not some sort of pregnancy slendertone, it is a big thick latex ball which promises not to burst (it can take up to 300 lb/21½ stone in weight) and tones the supportive muscles in your spine. Remember those fashionable gym shoes that cost a fortune? The ones based on the Masai tribe in Africa who were noted as having the best posture in the human race because they walked barefoot on uneven ground? Apparently having to correct your posture continually tightens up all those lazy leg muscles. The Gym or Birth Ball works on the same principle – just the act of staying on top of the ball while you are doing your make-up or watching telly, keeps you toned and 'helps your baby get into the optimal foetal position' by raising your hips higher than your knees. Besides, you can use it after the birth as a handy computer stool, as this typed sentence proves, and for bouncing your toddlers away from the keyboard as they sit on your knee swiping at it with sticky fingers.

For extroverts who want to bring it in to the hospital, may I just issue one word of warning. A friend Rosie fell pregnant in New York and could not get her birthing ball into the boot of the yellow cab as she contracted away on the pavement. In the end she sailed off to hospital leaving the blue spacehopper behind. Check your boot size, or inflate it once installed, before rolling in to hospital.

For the most comprehensive essay ever written on the benefits of a birth ball, visit (and buy) from www.activebirthcentre.com. At the time of writing it's yours for £29.95 plus pump.

Chung and Shake Those Apples

Because labour is all about trying to get you to relax so that the cervix will dilate, you can always show this page to your midwives ahead of time to ask whether they might be game for some way-out ways of helping labour progress.

For example, what our German friends call *die äpfel schüttelm* or 'shaking the apples' is a technique whereby the buttocks or thighs are jostled rhythmically as a way of softening up a mother's tension in the legs.

Alternatively, you could try to '*Chung*', a practice favoured in rural China. The labouring mother stands up, surrounded by her midwives, who then proceed to shake her vigorously. Despite the fact that it looks painful to the onlooker, one American midwife who observed Chunging in action said that the woman swore afterwards that it felt great.

Another firm favourite, which is a little less offbeam, is the **salsa dance**. This I witnessed in action on the Discovery Health Channel when a series called *Portland*

Babies ran in March 2004. There was a lovely moment during one birth when the midwives Fiona and Liz wanted to get labour going for a mother who seemed resigned to lie on her back. They showed her how to do the 'salsa dance' by standing with her feet a hip-width apart and rocking her hips from side to side. The midwives did it with her and within minutes the atmosphere in the room had changed from a downbeat to an upbeat one as everyone started giggling. The dancing really did get things going, and the mother still got to lie down, on her side, to birth her baby soon after.

Bottom Jokes

While we are firmly into our bodies, it is time to have a brief word about bottoms. Bottoms are useful things, because their workings can help us understand about what happens in labour. I was told by a friend who had an epidural birth that delivering a baby was like 'pushing a basketball out of your bum'. Certainly true if you are anaesthetized from the waist down and left guessing at how to get the baby out (not so if you are endorphined up to the eyeballs and your body is doing it for you).

Bottoms are particularly useful for teaching you about some of the reactions that you might experience during birth – a subject called 'Sphincter Law', and described by Ina May Gaskin in her *Guide to Childbirth*

(Random House, 2003). All sphincters, including the cervix and vagina, obey certain rules. In a nutshell, they are as follows:

a) sphincters function best in an atmosphere of familiarity and privacy
b) sphincters do not obey orders, such as 'Push!' or 'Just Relax!'
c) a person's sphincter in the process of opening may suddenly close down if that person becomes upset, frightened, humiliated or self-conscious
d) a relaxed mouth and jaw (laughing, singing, speaking loving words, telling bottom jokes or mooing are particularly recommended) is directly correlated to the ability of the cervix, vagina or anus to open to full capacity.

This last tenet of the law could be practised in the bathroom when next sitting on the pot home alone.

You only have to remember the last time you clamped up in the office loo when the boss walked in, or the last bout of constipation brought on by travelling through foreign towns with restrooms that you didn't want to visit, to know that Gaskin is right. 'According to Sphincter Law, labours that don't result in a normal birth after a "reasonable" amount of time are often slowed or stalled because of lack of privacy, fear and stimulation of the wrong part of the labouring woman's brain,' she writes. If you fear that Sphincter Law will not be respected in your chosen place of birth, perhaps it is wise investing in a Do-not-disturb sign or a bouncer at the door. Finally, when in labour, midwife Mary Cronk advises that **you remember the Four Fs: Feel Free to Fart Freely**.

4

Free Your Mind (and Your Ass Will Follow)

Working on your body is a lot easier than working on your mind. Having your foot massaged by a reflexologist or long fine needles put into your back are preferable to the worst sticky silence with a shrink. I spent three years on the couch in therapy (two and a half years more than I needed to, but it was just so great to get out of the house on my own for an hour) and I still approached the blue door every week with a sense of dread. The dread was fear of the unknown (what can of worms will I open today?) despite the fact that whenever I left, I came out feeling lighter, as though I had cleaned out my mental handbag.

Looking at your 'stuff' is not easy, and most of you probably equate psychotherapy with mild lunacy, so I am not about to advocate my particular (expensive, but cheap at the price) approach. The hardest part about starting therapy is, well, starting it. The second hardest part is finding a good recommended shrink, and stopping it is nigh on impossible. I cannot count how many sessions I had just talking about when I was going to stop. At least I got out before suffering the fate of one friend, however, who knew her time was up when she caught her shrink nodding off as she bared her heart.

If you are in therapy when you fall pregnant, you are in luck. You have a guaranteed space to process the huge change you are going through to become a mother. If you are not, and think shrinks are for mad people, then pregnancy is probably not the time to start anyway. Wait until you feel like murdering your husband, then you are ready.

Meditation and Visualization

One discipline that you can start while pregnant, that won't cost you anything and is perfectly safe, is a little meditation. It doesn't have to be done every day, just when you remember, and it may feel a little strange to do if you haven't done it before. The difficulty is in 'making your mind still' and not sitting there with your eyes closed distracted by the traffic outside or your things-to-do-list that keeps popping into your head. One friend, Isabella, who has just finished a course in Transcendental Meditation, said that she noticed in the first week how she hadn't shouted once at the children. 'Meditation gives you some control over your feelings, enabling you to deal with whatever is thrown at you,' she commented.

Sue Hollins, who teaches meditation courses in Brighton, recommends practising being still for 5 minutes every day while pregnant. 'Light a candle,' says Sue, 'which is a symbol of spiritual practice and has been used in church ceremonies in the West and the East down the ages, and place your feet on the ground. Pregnancy is such a special, sacred time, when you are bringing into the world new life that it is important to hold that and to be present in your body.'

Sue recommended to one of her pregnant students to visualize her baby in the womb, with the womb being the most beautiful place to be. Her student visualized her baby lying on pillows made of angel wings, with blossom falling all around. Towards the end of her pregnancy, when she had problems sleeping, she went on to visualize herself in the same place, and her sleeping improved.

Visualization and affirmations are also used in labour to help women stay calm and focused. Some prefer to use a mantra that they have practised in meditation, while others find a single word or phrase such as 'release', 'open up' or 'let go' to be useful.

In the book *Healthy Body, Better Birthing* (Newleaf, 2001), the authors Francesca Naish and Janette Roberts suggest imagining your cervix as a flower opening up in time-lapse photography, or surfing waves as an analogy for contractions. They recommend some of the following mantras for the last stages of pregnancy and during the birth: 'I embrace the intensity of birth'; 'the birth of my baby is a miracle of life'; 'I will make my needs clear to others'; 'I am open to the best possible birth'; 'I trust in my strength.'

If repeating the above is just going to make you giggle, or start talking in an American accent, try nothing more than just listening to your breath as you sit still for 5 minutes. 'The passage of oxygen into your body is like new life pouring in,' says Sue Hollins. 'As you exhale, breathe out the carbon dioxide, tiredness and worry that your body no longer wants to hold.' Ahhhhh.

Control Freaks

Talking to the American midwife Elizabeth Gilmore in New Mexico, I learned one professional's view about how an older mother differs from a younger mother: 'It's much easier to have a baby when a woman is young – not because of her body age, but because an older woman is used to being in control. Once you are 30 and you've been an executive and you've run your own household, and you're used to people doing what you say when you say, you have control. Then, at birth, you have to be prepared to give it all up,' says Gilmore. 'Young girls when they give birth are not used to control,' she continued, 'they are used to not being able to control anything and give it up quicker. But an older woman who is used to having things her way, and takes an aspirin when she has a headache, now has to go into a new space that she is not used to. That she left behind in childhood.'

Mmmm, loss of control. Tough one for us stiff-upper-lip Brits. Gilmore is not talking about losing control over how you want the birth to go here, she's talking about the very visceral side of giving birth, the last contractions when the body wants to do its job and needs its owner to just let go and let it. Not unlike the orgasm analogy again. Or as the New Zealanders at the Common Knowledge Trust say, 'birth is learning to control surrender'.

It's a grey area, letting go of our feelings and exploring what it is *we really want*. There is always plenty of talk by politicians about 'women being given enough information to make "informed choices"' in maternity matters, but there are thousands of women who want someone else to make up their minds for them. Many of us would prefer to be good little girls, approved of by those around us, not making a noise or a fuss, and are socially conditioned to do what the midwives and doctors tell us. All others want is safe delivery of a healthy baby, and some almost give up on their own good health to achieve it. Once you have had a baby, however, you realize how instrumental your own wellbeing is for caring for that demanding little terrorist, sorry, adorable little newborn.

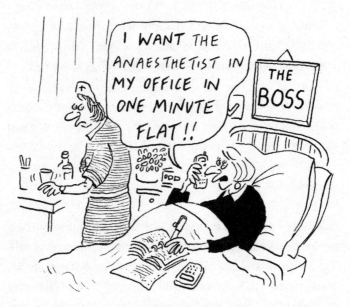

Who Am I, and Do I Exist?

With freedom of choice comes responsibility, and responsibility is a big one. There is a big payoff, however. Exploring the matter of your birth is all about preparation for motherhood, and what you learn about yourself on the way will have a much greater impact on your mothering than any amount of NCT classes.

Don't rely on your husband, doctor or midwife to make the decisions for you, or give up by announcing 'We'll see what happens on the day.' Make a pact with yourself and the baby to do it for the both of you. As Eminem says, 'You only get one chance!' You were looking after your unborn baby long before you had even met the midwife and obstetrician, and you will be in it together long after their names slip your mind. In our baby-centred culture, where mothers are seen as little more than vessels for bringing forth the all-important child, you may have to refuse to be cajoled into something you don't want or, God forbid, go elsewhere if you don't feel you're being listened to. The strength you gain from speaking your truth now, however shy and timid you normally are, will help you be a more confident mother. You may even suffer disapproval from others with your choices. Unpopular? Me? But I get along with everybody and am so easy to please! Just wait until you board an aircraft with your fractious baby – then you will know about unpopularity. Indeed, learning to weather occasional unpopularity is an extremely useful parenting skill in this country.

No More Ms Nice Guy

The great thing about taking responsibility for your birth is that you don't blame anyone else if things don't go according to plan. So, you wanted a drug-free birth, and you changed your mind in labour and had an epidural. Fine, you can look back on your birth and feel happy that you still felt in charge and listened to, and you did the best you could. However, if someone else pressurizes you to take that decision, and you thought you were doing OK, just needed more time, then your feelings about the birth might be mixed. At best you will slowly come round to the view that perhaps it was the right decision in the circumstances; at worst you will remember that aspect of the birth above all others, and the birth will play over and over in your mind like a broken video cassette.

For example, if you haven't looked into whether you want to go for an epidural (bearing in mind it means less mobility in labour, and therefore a higher likelihood of giving birth on your back with an episiotomy and stitches to follow, then you may find yourself in a tug-of-war between the midwives and the doctors on the day. Cristina Odone, deputy editor of the *New Statesman*, described this scenario in a Radio Four

Woman's Hour special on birth broadcast in November 2003:

When I went into my NHS flagship hospital for an induction, I was told that if I was worried [about the strong and often more painful contractions that follow an induction] I could have an epidural. When the doctor left the room the midwives said, 'It's so much preferable if you can have a natural birth, it is much the best way.' I might have been swayed if it hadn't been for my wonderful partner Edward who had been there and was very protective and said 'But you said you wanted an epidural if it becomes a very painful ordeal.' It was as if the medics and the midwives were playing for a power struggle in who was more powerful, and I was just a pawn in their game.

By being reminded of what she wanted by a supportive partner, Cristina was able to weather that tug-of-war. If you put yourself in charge now during pregnancy, and that includes getting the right birth partner to support you on the day (see page 78), you will be in the right frame of mind to decide for yourself and the baby on the right course for labour. That doesn't mean that you can't change your mind about what you want in the middle of it, but it does mean that you won't feel like a victim when circumstances takes a different course. Make a pact with yourself now, say 'I'm in charge of my baby, and will be for many years to come, not the doctors and midwives. They are only here to help and give advice.'

Yeah, Right. Get a Life.

My overly long time in therapy spanned my second pregnancy with the twins and was a great support through the difficult last stage when I was fighting with the NHS to get the birth I wanted. My shrink was an older mother figure, who parried my best attempts for direction by asking. 'Aha, you are trying to make me give you the answers again, it is not about what *I* want, it is about what *you* want.' Sometimes she'd catch herself doling out maternal advice until she'd stop and announce how well I'd managed to manipulate her into doing all the talking again, when the answer had to come from me. 'What do I feel about this?' became my mantra as I started a big information-gathering exercise about the best steps to take.

My therapist supported me through all of this, and yet was always pushing me a little harder to go a little deeper. My views felt validated by her listening to me, which is often all women need to gain confidence in themselves. Once the long process of exploring what I wanted was over, acting upon it was fairly quick.

The sort of therapy I was in used different techniques to draw out difficult customers. Sometimes we'd use role-play to work through problems, sometimes we used drawing. As someone who could only draw stick people, it was fun to get the crayons out and not be inhibited about careless colouring. I was always amazed at how differently the drawings were interpreted by another to how I perceived my state of mind. At one moment I thought I was fairly relaxed in my family life, and then the sketch of a cage with rows of gnashing teeth suggested something otherwise.

Draw Out Those Fears

Drawing played a big part in the Art of Birthing Classes, described to me by the midwife Elizabeth Gilmore in New Mexico, and charted in Pamela England's book *Birthing from Within* (Partera Press, 1998). I read a beaten-up copy while sitting in the American Birth Centre under a psychedelic painting of a mother cradling her newborn with fireworks exploding around her. As Gilmore describes:

We'd look for examples in the pregnant woman of where they have this incredible strength, and help them learn to use that strength to tolerate pain and lack of control. We did a lot of work with art and clay and drumming and singing to help women find the 'tiger within'. She [Pamela England] had the idea of exploring who are you: what are your fears, what are your strengths and doing that with art – looking at birth as a vision quest: you are going to go through death of your former self and go through trial by fire, to achieve something so magnificent as the safe bringing of a child.

Now, making a 'belly cast' out of paper-mâché of your huge boobs and stomach in the last weeks of pregnancy may not be your idea of an average NCT class ('It's great for dips 'n' chips' announced one romantic father, while another couple lay a sheepskin rug inside the belly cast to use as a Moses basket when the baby arrived). However, the drawing exercises and art therapy documented in *Birthing from Within* worked on a deep level for many of the women in the book. To my knowledge, no birth workshops exist like this in the UK. But anyone interested in exploring the meaning of their doodles further could do worse than buy the book or visit the website where suggestions for finding workshops are given: www.birthingfromwithin.com.

Neurotics Rule, um, OK?

While talking birth stories with Sue Hollins, a counsellor and mother of three teenagers, Sue had the realization that while her first two pregnancies were wonderful, and she walked around in some sort of happy daze, untouched by the cares of the world and floating above it all, her first two labours were not so out of this world. During her pregnancy with her third child, her back gave way as she shouldered more and more responsibility for the family without asking for help or support. The back crisis forced her in late pregnancy to put herself first. Despite her physical handicap, her last birth was the easiest of all three.

Phoebe entered the world with a few pushes, to be caught just in time by her father. Sue reflected that those who have easy and relaxed pregnancies by no means go on to have easy and relaxed births. Indeed, perhaps the opposite was true. Those who were fearful and a little anxious, grounded in the real world, were more likely to be realistic and present during the birth.

In the next few interviews for birth stories with women who had exceptionally good births, I tried out the theory, which certainly chimed with my own experience. In my first birth I sailed through pregnancy and loved it, and accepted unquestioningly every medical intervention in the book. Afterwards, I felt as if I had been run over by a bus and didn't go outside for the first two weeks. With my second pregnancy, when I found out at 30 weeks that I had a struggle on my hands to get the birth I wanted, I suddenly snapped out of my cosy pregnancy stupor and woke up to the potential nightmare ahead. Many of the birth stories in the next chapter include some form of awakening, or reality check, that focused these women on their birth and helped them to go on to birth well.

In *Birthing from Within*, psychologist Dr Lewis Mehl talks about a childbirth class in Georgia, US that he visited. One of the six couples in the class was obsessed with details of a Caesarean birth and how to avoid it, stretching the patience of their childbirth teacher as each week they came in with fresh questions requiring fresh answers. Later, at a reunion after the births, everyone was amazed that the couple who had worried so much about the Caesarean had birthed normally, while every other couple in the class had a Caesarean birth. **Mehl concluded afterwards that 'Worry was the work of pregnancy.'**

Airing any concerns that you have over the birth and what may happen, particularly to someone who is emotionally supportive of you – including the midwife who might be attending you on the day – is more likely to reduce your anxiety levels than increase them. Don't let these worries become little nattering devils in the back of your mind – write them down, make a list, and get them out in the open. My big fear in planning a home birth with my twins was that if medical help was needed, I would be too far from the hospital. When I told my midwife about this, she explained to me that the main reason why women transfer to hospital during labour at home is because it progresses too slowly, not too fast. I was only partially satisfied.

At the next meeting, I told her that I was still a little anxious over this matter, and she went on to explain NHS procedures. She told me how, if an ambulance were called, I would be viewed as an emergency case with all doctors and anaesthetists on call waiting at the door for me to be 'bluelighted' into the hospital. Therefore, as they were obliged to be there, I would get better treatment than if I were already in hospital, when the doctor might be attending another birth, the anaesthetist might be in the canteen and the extra midwife on her tea break, all of them grumbling to their pagers: 'OK, we'll be along in a minute.' That reassured me, as did the story of an even more neurotic home-birth woman who called an ambulance anyway when she went into labour, and got her mother to ply the paramedics with biscuits and cups of tea until the birth was over.

It seems that the best course in pregnancy is to address your fears as early as possible and out them. Don't be patronized by people who say, 'Don't worry, everything will be fine.' Find someone who will listen properly and answer you truthfully until you feel satisfied. If you are still confused, keep asking – birth is a very complicated subject and you may need to find a specialist to help you to understand. If you don't, those worries may surface again in labour and slow, or even halt altogether, the process. As Carl Jung wrote, 'With knowledge, the unconscious is robbed of its fire.'

Little White Pills for the Mind

If talking just isn't your style, try homoeopathy. Homoeopathy is the kind of subject that sends my husband, an unreconstructed Yorkshireman, down the pub for a game of dominos. He'd argue that it works because of the placebo effect, but the many, like myself, who have found it helpful in 'restoring the body to a state of balance by adding minute amounts of what you are lacking' would argue otherwise. The theory is that those minute amounts of 'energy medicine' stimulate the body's natural resources to produce what is missing, thus putting your body back into a state of harmony.

As well as the little bags of pills that you take home, the act of sitting in a room with a homoeopath has its own healing effect, as you are questioned about your sleeping, eating and emotional state in an insightful way that makes you feel strangely validated. (This relationship is good to set up now, because you are likely to return with a baby or toddler in tow when their own coughs, colds or rashes need an alternative approach.)

In labour and birth, homoeopathy is found to be so useful that many independent midwives use it. Talking to Caroline Gaskin, a homoeopath who specializes in homoeopathy for pregnancy and birth at the Active Birth Centre in north London, she tells me that as well as helping women who are warned off conventional medicine during pregnancy, she also makes up specific remedies for pain-management in labour. Because of the nature of birth, the remedies tend to be in a 'high energetic potency'. 'I always tell women that there will be two things likely to happen in their birth, that it will be tiring and it will be painful, and then I give them the remedies to support these two processes.'

For this, Arnica tends to be the key remedy. 'Beyond that, there are two areas where problems can occur,' continues Caroline. 'The first tends to be emotional, when the labour is slowed down for some. And secondly, for the physical reason that the contractions are inefficient – where there is too much pain and not enough action.' She offers different remedies based on the underlying cause. 'For a labour that is stopping and starting, I might use Pulsatilla, or for low Braxton Hicks [tightening around the stomach as the body limbers up for labour] or to help with early labour pains, I might suggest Caullophyllum.' She also says, 'I am often asked by women if there are any remedies to induce labour, but homoeopathy cannot be used to cause a push/shove effect. If a woman is overdue and anxious, I might suggest reflexology or acupuncture.'

Caroline Gaskin often sees women towards the end of their pregnancy, and recommends the Yellow Childbirth Kit (see below) as a good way of familiarizing yourself with the different remedies before going into labour. 'The great thing about homoeopathy is that if it doesn't work, there is no harm done. Because it is an energy medicine, you can't take too much – in fact most people need to repeat the remedy and take it more often rather than less,' says Caroline, who does workshops with doulas (see page 80) and offers to email anyone interested with specific information on homoeopathic remedies for labour and postnatal healing: CarolineGaskin@blueyonder.co.uk.

To find a registered homoeopath in your area, contact the Alliance of Registered Homoeopaths (www.a-r-h.org). To self-prescribe, you can buy a Yellow Childbirth Kit direct from the Helios Homoeopathic Pharmacy for £26.95 (www.helios.co.uk, tel. 01892 537254). If you do decide to go this route, your birth partner also needs to be familiar with the remedies, in case, for example, you need a remedy for being in a state of denial. For further reading, see *The Women's Guide to Homoeopathy* by Dr Andrew Lockie and Dr Nicola Geddes (Hamish Hamilton).

5

Can You Feel It?

Emotion n. *Any strong feeling, as of joy, sorrow, or fear* (16C from Latin, *emovere*, **to disturb**) – *Collins English Dictionary*

This is the chapter that nearly didn't get written. Being a casualty of boarding school, sent away at 10, I used to deal with my feelings by keeping them locked away like sweets in a tuck box. A great survival tactic when away from your mother, but not useful when you are about to become one. In pregnancy, when you are swimming in a sea of hormones, it is impossible not to be emotional most of the time. When a baby is growing inside, you are vulnerable to a whole new way of thinking and being, which may be an enhancement of your already sensitive nature or, in my case, a holiday from your emotionally-constipated one.

While I was pregnant, I didn't make any decision – small or large – until I had asked myself 'What do I feel about this?' It was as much the novelty of asking this question and getting an answer, a change from my usual indecisiveness, that prompted my questioning. I so enjoyed the sensation of knowing what I felt about things all the time, that I allowed my feelings to govern the course of my pregnancy (poor husband).

So much for the positive aspect of feelings that let you tap into your true nature and take responsibility for your actions. But what of the negative side, such as fear and loathing, which can also dictate the way you behave? Some women become so terrified about the thought of giving birth when pregnant, usually because of previous trauma, that they are medically classified as *partumphobics*. For them we must be thankful that the National Health System still supports a woman's right to choose, if choosing to be anaesthetized and having a Caesarean birth is the way they want to go. For the rest of us, it is a question of Feeling the Fear and Doing it Anyway. And for this, one of the greatest props we can have is Emotional Support.

Guardian Angels

Husband, partner, doula, independent midwife, yoga teacher, mother, friend, relative – your birth partners are your first defence against fear. While you have the job of birthing the baby, they are your support system (sometimes there to be leaned on, literally) and your emotional prop. If you want to have more than one prop, then you are quite within your rights to do so.

Just recently, the Government report on Choice in Maternity Services announced, 'We do not think it is reasonable that women should be limited to a single birth partner in any circumstances. Such an attitude suggests birth is being managed for the convenience of the unit rather than the mother. We look to the Department [of Health] to support the view that women should not be limited to a single birth partner.' There. The PM has personally OKed the presence of your husband *and* your mother in the delivery suite.

Emotional support comes best from someone who knows you well and believes in you, and is different from the professional support you might get from a midwife. As the midwife Fiona explains in the series *Portland Babies*: 'If you can find someone to come in who is in tune with the woman in labour, then this can really help things along. Their additional emotional support is different from the care we give as midwives.'

Hopeless Husbands and Perfect Partners

Emotions may dictate whom we want at the birth. Unusually for today, my husband did not want to be there for my labour, preferring instead to come in immediately afterwards to meet his sons and daughter. After my initial disappointment I respected his decision, knowing that a part of me would be looking after *him* during labour ('Darling, oweeeeeee, you look bored … why don't you pop down to the shop for a newspaper?'). I also harboured secret worries that he would react badly to all my huffing and puffing, would be traumatized by the gore or, worst of all, would only listen to the doctor's ideas about what should be happening instead of mine. He would assume his mantle of a professional lawyer talking to a professional doctor, and I would be waving my hand in opposition between them while having a contraction.

To make up for his absence I needed to find emotional support from elsewhere (a best friend at the first birth, my mother at the second) to help me through. **You cannot afford to have anyone at your birth who may be looking to *you* for emotional support**. It can only work the other way round. If your partner fits into my category, think about having someone else there *as well as him* to relieve the burden. With hindsight, not having my husband Adam there until he walked in after the birth had an unexpected bonus: he was able to meet his babies fresh as a daisy, bonding with all three of them beautifully for hours while I slept in the corner like some exhausted old drunk.

Only you and your partner can discuss this thorny issue of who will be doing what on the day, and your own fears may play a part in the discussion. It was only a generation ago that men were actively discouraged from attending a birth, and my mother talks about how women feared that they would be 'robbed of their mystery' if the father witnessed the act.

The modern view is wholly different. Theatre Director Dominic Dromgoole, a keen attendant at all three of his daughters' births (see Water Birth at Home, page 129) says, 'How any man could think that the mystery would be blown away by watching a fully-formed baby emerging is beyond me. I mean, it's not like they're doing a poo, is it? They're creating a little cathedral of a human being, which is the most complex and extraordinary mechanism that nature has yet evolved. So, if anything, it increases your admiration for what that already mysterious cavity is capable of. It's not as if men are endowed with such extraordinary orifices anyway.' Dominic also points out that, with so much action going on, you don't stop to think, '"Oh, lord what is happening to my wife's beautiful jewel?" – The two processes are completely separate.'

It is certainly true that, for some men, without advice from their own fathers who were relegated to the pub for the birth, they do find it difficult knowing how to act. Dominic had been given some advice about establishing boundaries in the hospital early on, and followed it to the letter. 'Someone had told me that it's important to establish that the hospital room belongs to you and your partner having a baby – not the hospital.' When the midwife came in and asked Dominic to move his bag on arrival, he 'had a little spat with her', reminding her whose room it was and that they could put their things where they liked. 'There's so much turf war going on in hospitals anyway, it's important to stake your claim early on. It was very different for our second birth at home, where it was very much *our* territory and people were invited in to *our* house and stuck to *our* rules.'

Choosing a Birth Partner

If you have someone other than your partner, you need to consider two things: do they have faith in a normal birth process (my best friend had had two normal births before assisting me)? And, are you reasonably unselfconscious with them (have they heard you swear recently)? It's not that in the throes of labour you will turn into some wailing witch with mad hair – people forget that **labour is often an expression of who you are, so shy people tend to have quiet births, while extroverts tend to show off a bit** – it's just that any hidden reservations need to be outed with that person BEFORE you go into labour. If they aren't, they may interfere with the birth process. Whomever you choose, promise me one thing. **Don't even think about doing it on your own. Hospitals are brutal places and you need someone to hold your hand, and anybody is better than nobody**. Especially if that anybody is a strong type, happy to approach a desk of chattering nurses or chivvy along absent midwives. If you can find someone who makes you laugh as well, then you may not even need gas and air.

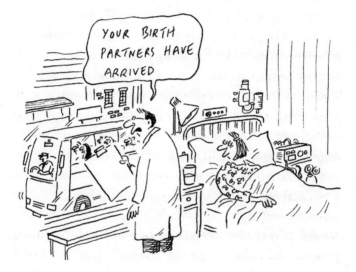

Go Doolally and Hire a Doula

A modern and successful addition to the Emotional Support Team is a doula. In the book *Mothering the Mother* (Da Capo Press), one father comments 'I've run a number of marathons, I've done a lot of hiking with a heavy backpack, and I've worked for 40 hours straight on call; but going through labour with my wife was more strenuous and exhausting than any of these experiences.' And this was from a man who had a doula with him. Because supporting a wife in labour can be particularly draining for a husband or partner because of their emotional involvement (having to deal with seeing a partner in pain, fearing for the outcome for the child), the rise in the number of doulas to relieve partners in labour has taken off in the last 10 years.

Doula (Greek for 'female slave', and not the more politically-correct translation 'woman caregiver') is the missing link between our ancestors' experience of giving birth with an experienced woman at her side, and our modern route of relying on technology and husbands to see us through. A doula is not a doctor, nurse or midwife with any training in medical matters, but is experienced in childbirth and has learned about medical interventions so that she can explain them to parents during labour.

As well as having your partner, the value of having an independent emotional support during labour is 'priceless', as one mother describes. Anita Lewisohn had a 'traumatic' first birth after being induced at Kingston Hospital in Surrey. She felt ignored as the hospital were short of staff and went into full-blown labour suddenly and painfully. Second time around she hired a doula, went into labour spontaneously on her due date and says,

I'd have probably been all right without a doula, but the added reassurance she brought me was priceless. I just felt that I had someone completely on my side who knew the ropes and had seen it all before.

For every contraction, she massaged my back really hard, which helped a lot, then brought me sips of water and was incredibly attentive to my every need in a way that my husband Al, wonderful though he is, would never have thought of doing. So Al basically held my hand (very tight) while she was much more active in helping me through it, along with a very young midwife.

A study done in Houston, Texas proved the value of a doula's continual emotional support for a woman in labour.[1] Women entering the Jefferson Davis Hospital in 1987 were offered a doula to support them during labour as part of a study. Out of the 416 women participating, roughly half agreed to have an unknown doula, as well as a friend and family member visiting, if the labour room was not too busy during their birth. By way of background to the study, it is worth knowing that birth is highly medicalized in the States, and was particularly so back in the 1980s. Most 'patients' were confined to bed, had an electronic foetal monitor attached, and had their waters broken at 5cm so another foetal monitor could be attached to the baby's scalp. Labour was expected to follow a set pattern, and oxytocin was given if labour was not progressing fast enough.

In the doula group the labours of the women averaged 7.4 hours, while in the no-doula group they lasted 9.4 hours on average. In the doula group 55 per cent of the women birthed 'normally' (with no anaesthesia, oxytocin, medication or forceps); in the no-doula group only 12 per cent achieved this. Perhaps the most interesting variation was in the demand for epidural pain-relief. In the no-doula group, 55 per cent of women asked for one, while only 8 per cent of the doula group did the same. The mothers in the doula group had never met nor expected to receive this kind of support, and yet the doulas' presence, along with their verbal support 'offering comfort, reassurance and praise' directly affected these women's experiences of birth.

The accompaniment of a doula can also be beneficial in other ways. Expecting your husband or partner to turn into a caring, sharing Florence Nightingale overnight can put a lot of expectation and strain on your relationship. Many fathers (but not all) welcome the presence of an extra pair of hands; it helps them to relax and feel that they are not shouldering all the responsibility for the labour (as if that were the case). Others like to have an excuse to nod off in the corner of the room or answer their mobile. My own dear brother, who coached the last Women's Modern Pentathlon Olympic team to medal victory in Athens, cheering them through their five races of running, riding, swimming, fencing and shooting, still managed to conk out during his own wife's long labour, snoring away on a chair. Unsurprisingly, for baby number two, he was not the only labour coach invited along.

There is one further study done with doulas, which goes a long way towards explaining the value of getting birth right. This study, in Johannesburg, looked at the postpartum health of mothers who were looked after during their birth by doulas. At six weeks after the birth, 59 per cent of the women who had chosen to birth with doulas were still breastfeeding their babies, while only 29 per cent of the no-doula group were. Mothers supported by doulas also reported feeling twice as satisfied in their relationship with their partners after the birth as those who did not hire a doula. The no-doula group, meanwhile, responded to a questionnaire saying that their babies had nearly double the number of coughs, colds, runny noses, poor appetites and diarrhoea as the doula group – when there was no difference in the mothers' health on admission to hospital.[2] The authors of the book *Mothering the Mother*,

Marshall and Phyllis Klaus and John Kennell, ask 'Can the presence of a doula during labour reduce a mother's anxiety sufficiently and give her such a boost in self-esteem that she considers her baby to be healthier?'

If you can afford to pay for a doula to answer this question, then consider it money well spent. Doulas, most of whom have to have a Doula qualification to call themselves such nowadays, can be found via Nanny Agencies in the Yellow Pages or through an organization called Doula UK (www.doula.org.uk) which helps people find a doula locally without an agency charge.

Bond with Me, Baby

In *A Life's Work* (Fourth Estate), Rachel Cusk writes on recovering from her Caesarean birth:

It is as if I am unable to find any connection between my physical implication in the fact of her [the baby's] existence, and the emotional world I had imagined would automatically accompany it, a world in which I would automatically be included.

Pregnancy begins to seem to me more and more of a lie, a place populated by evangelicals and moralists and control-freaks, a place haunted by crazies with their delusions of motherhood. Or perhaps it is the clinical, hospital-appointed nature of the birth itself that has caused me to lose the thread of things, for in truth my experience of birth was more like the experience of having an appendix removed than what most people would understand by 'labour'. Without its connecting hours, the glue of its pain, the literalness of its passage, I fear that I will not make it to motherhood; that I will remain stranded as someone who merely had an operation, leaving the baby with no more sense of how she came to be here than if she had been left on the doorstep by a stork.

Images of Madonna and Child, mother and baby entwined in an eternal embrace of love may have fuelled your expectations of motherhood, but bonding is not always Love at First Sight. The books might say that it can take days or weeks to bond with your child, but for many it may be months or years until they gaze at their little boy or girl in the park and feel that pure outpouring of love that announces that There Is No Going Back. This is worth remembering now, because you don't want to beat yourself up or harbour secret worries about whether 'it' has happened yet, in those early days after the birth. **Just be sure that it will happen, because it will**. And making sure that you are properly supported around the birth is one of the best ways of helping it to happen earlier rather than later.

For Jenny, who was left alone for most of her first labour and had a standard medicalized birth, the removal of her baby immediately after the birth caused her unfounded anxiety. Her daughter was not returned until some time later, and Jenny worried in the meantime that there were problems with the baby. At nine years old, her daughter Elizabeth began to make critical comments about Jenny's failure to cuddle or touch her. Jenny recognized that her attitude towards her daughter was probably the reason for Elizabeth's attention-seeking behaviour, which was becoming more and more inappropriate as she was nearing puberty. Jenny sought help from Beverley Beech at the Association for Improvements in the Maternity Services (AIMS) about her birth experience, and it was suggested that she talk to Elizabeth about it. The moment came when they were doing some embroidery together, when Jenny began to tell Elizabeth about the difficulties she felt around the birth. Mother and daughter cried together afterwards, and comforted each other with hugs.

Beverley Beech reported in *Midwifery Digest*: 'Since then Jenny found the change in her daughter remarkable. No longer was she seeking attention from anyone who visited the house, and, even better, Jenny found that her reluctance to cuddle and touch her daughter had evaporated.' Beech concludes: 'With good, kindly and supportive midwifery care even those mothers who have had difficult, stressful and traumatic labours, some of which end up with caesarean sections, report they can look back on the births positively because of the quality of support, respect and kindness they experienced.'[3]

Way back in 1976, studies done by Marshall Klaus and John Kennell showed that interference with the normal bonding process has a great and sometimes drastic impact on the family.[4] Current hospital practice has incorporated some of their findings, and today the period immediately after the birth is recognized as important, with mothers offered skin-to-skin contact with their babies and left undisturbed with the fathers for a while. Mothers who are given this time of grace are known to hold their babies more competently, establish more intimate contact with them and to have fewer problems with breastfeeding than those who are separated from their children.

Klaus and Kennell's later analysis of women supported by doulas during labour chime with Beverley Beech's views about the importance of qualities such as kindness and respect during the process. There were no differences in hospital admissions between the doula and no-doula group, and yet when the mothers were asked how much time they spent away from their babies in a week, and the number of days it had taken to develop a significant relationship, the differences were significant. Mothers in the doula group said they spent 1.7 hours a week away from their baby, in contrast to the no-doula mothers who were away 6.6 hours. The doula group said it took on average 2.9 days to develop a relationship with their babies, compared to 9.8 days for the other group of mothers.[5] Klaus and Kennell suggest 'Such striking differences ... from such a short period of support is a reminder that the period of labour is a time when the mother is especially sensitive to environmental factors and open to learning and growth.' [6]

And if you are looking for the best professional support available to a woman in labour, you need look no further than independent midwives.

Independent Midwives: Angels without Wings

If there is anything slightly high-risk or complicated about your birth, or you want 'continuity of care' and you can afford the additional cost, then independent midwives are the Rolls-Royce of birth assistants. They might even provide the answer to our flagging NHS maternity services if all of them out there were given a contract to practise alongside hospital midwives and boost numbers. Not only would they help make up for the current shortage, but they would also inject real skill and experience into the business. If current lobbying from the Independent Midwives Association goes ahead, it may yet happen.

In the meantime, we can count our lucky stars that independent midwives are still with us and haven't been driven away by a nasty insurance clause that their statutory body, the Nursing and Midwifery Council, nearly inserted into their code of practice in 2003. Because independent midwives cannot afford to practise with full indemnity insurance (no insurance company will insure them for what they do), they have always relied on informing their clients about the impossibility of suing them should anything happen over the birth. As the most common reason for suing any institution or medical practitioner is 'negligence', and the words 'independent midwife' and 'negligent' don't sit happily in the same sentence, the issue very rarely occurs. However, the NMC – in attempting to clarify this insurance matter – threatened to wipe out the practice of independent midwives for good. Fortunately a deluge of letters in their support from women who had been attended by these guardian angels, and some strong politicking in Parliament, kept them in business. Lucky for you, should you decide to hire one.

My own independent midwife, Mary Cronk, is one of the most experienced in the country, a founder of the Association of Radical Midwives, and in her early days flew all over the country to deliver babies for women at home. Knowing that she had delivered well over 100 sets of twins in her time gave me utter reassurance in her ability, and her experience gave me confidence that I could birth my twins normally. Having Mary and another independent midwife, Andrea Dombrowe (independent midwives work in pairs and cover for each other), with me as I walked into hospital made me feel like I was entering hospital with two Roman centurions at my side. Ain't nobody gonna mess with them. And when the hospital midwife did come in to announce that she was in charge, Mary reminded her quite firmly that, 'Actually, my client is in charge here.' All empowering stuff. As the first baby's head crowned and this voice came from within me growling, 'Bloody hell, that hurts,' I was only aware of Mary's voice of encouragement. She gave me total faith that I could do it. And it all went so well, largely thanks to her.

Most independent midwives belong to the Independent Midwives Association (IMA). Other experienced independent midwives in the south of the country from whom I have heard similarly ecstatic tales include Jane Evans and Val Taylor in Brighton. As well as helping at the birth, independent midwives do all your antenatal checks at home (except scans) and look after you for as much postpartum care as you need. All for around £2,500. For further information, phone 01483 821104, visit www.independentmidwives.org or send an s.a.e. to 1 The Great Quarry, Guildford GU1 3XL.

Come Hypnobirth with Me

If you don't feel you need that level of additional support, but are looking for something beyond the parentcraft classes to include your partner more in the experience, then the latest American import may be the answer to your prayers. Especially as the one course that

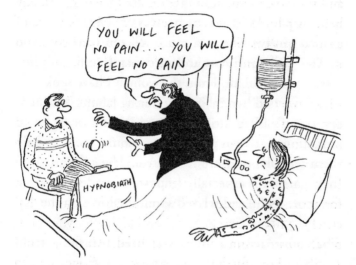

I researched in Northamptonshire cost around £200 for four classes, encompassing 10 hours' worth of teaching.

An American woman named Marie Mongan came up with hypnobirthing, and started training instructors in Britain in her techniques two years ago. In short, **she teaches people to rid themselves of the fear of pain, and to put women in a more relaxed state of mind so they feel confident and in control, and look forward to their birth**. From the women I have spoken to who have used hypnobirthing during labour (see Lindsey Lloyd's birth story, page 147), one of its main attractions is that it gives women some 'tools' to help them feel like they are in control. The support from their partner is especially important, and helps them feel more useful and relaxed about their role on the day.

The course teaches four specialized breathing techniques during which the birth partner is taught how to hypnotize the labouring woman and to do relaxation exercises with her. Before you get images of Paul McKenna performing wizardry with a glamorous assistant, the hypnosis is not so much putting you under as teaching you 'fear-release' and 'hypnoanaesthesia' – a form of numbing relaxation with tapes and music used as props. Apparently, having practised the relaxation exercises to the tapes, you find in labour that the music triggers the same response in the body, even when in such a heightened state.

Jenny Mullan, a teacher of the method in Northampton, claims that out of 10 women she has helped, all 10 birthed well as a result of the course – most needing no pain-relief at all. The two that I spoke to were evangelical in their praise of the method, both birthing in hospital without any pain-relief at all, and both admitting to feeling 'proud of themselves' for having a birth that went so well. To find a local practitioner in the UK, and to find out more about it, visit www.hypnobirth.info. The books and the tapes are only available as part of the course, and are not published in the UK, although *Hypnobirthing* can be bought as an imported book from amazon.com.

6

Away with the Fairies

None of us comes to birth as a stranger to pain. We may think of pain in terms of physical pain, but what about all the emotional pain we experience in our everyday lives such as fear, anger, grief or guilt, or mental pain in the form of negative thoughts that haunt us and make us unhappy? In fact, by the time we get to childbirth the only pain we may have yet to experience is 'positive' pain, the stretching of muscles to announce the arrival of new life – **a little bit of suffering for a sacred rite** of passage. That is one pain in the ass worth bearing.

The Point of Pain

There is a popular analogy that makes the rounds of antenatal classes that says 'If you were to go to the dentist to get a tooth pulled, you'd expect to have pain-relief. So why not do the same for childbirth?' It seems flawlessly logical, and suggests that women trying to birth without pain-relief are some cult of masochistic martyrs. Sadly, what the analogy misses out is that when birthing, pain is an essential part of the feedback loop for the mother. For example, if your contractions are getting stronger and you feel the need to get up and walk around to make them more bearable, then that is probably what your body needs to do at that moment to get the baby into a better position. Without the pain there would be no urge to move, and therefore no motivation to position the baby better.

In second stage, when you are pushing the baby out, the pain – which peaks for a maximum of a few contractions when the baby's head appears (called 'crowning' or, more accurately, 'ring of fire') – actually speeds up the whole process. It makes sense that if this is a painful job, your body wants to get on with it. The pain-feedback loop means that nerves in the cervix, pelvic floor muscles and vagina transmit stretching sensations to the pituitary gland which in turns produce more oxytocin, which in turns increases the speed of labour. If you can feel the pain, it is more likely to be over quickly.

This was certainly borne out by my own experience. With my first baby, after an epidural I spent *two hours* on my back pushing. I remember thinking to myself that labour was more like a long cross-country run than the sublime welcoming of a new life into the world. With hindsight, because the pain-feedback loop had been broken by the anaesthetic, I couldn't even feel my legs, let alone a contraction, and I needed synthetic oxytocin to be given through a drip to strengthen the contractions to keep labour going. Birth was a strange, disembodied experience, I only knew when to push because the pads on my stomach announced on the monitor the beginning of a contraction, and the two midwives watching the monitor would shout: 'Push!' Eventually I needed an episiotomy [snip] to birth my first son, Humphrey, who was born sideways like so many epidural babies, because he, too, could feel nothing but relaxed and flabby muscles to turn against.

Second time around, those few minutes through the 'ring of fire' with the twins – which seemed no worse than the 'Chinese burns' we used to give each other in the playground – were easily forgotten through the haze of endorphins and gas and air that saw me through. The next day I sat in the bath with my body feeling spookily back to normal, in spite of the fact that I had given birth only 24 hours earlier. What a difference from my first birth when, after the epidural and episiotomy, I spent two weeks dreading every trip to the bathroom, unable to sit anywhere comfortably with a body that would clamp up with pain performing the most basic bodily functions. The epidural birth may have been painless, but the discomfort afterwards was far worse than crowning for a few moments endorphined up to the eyeballs. Unsurprisingly, after a C-section – major abdominal surgery – it can be even worse. My friend Rosie's morphine drip was turned off by mistake on day two, and she likened it to 'someone stamping on my stomach with hobnailed boots'.

Nature's High

The good news is that nature has devised a miraculous way of dealing with all this pain, without any need to resort to hard drugs. When you think 300,000 women are giving birth all over the world on any given day, many of them in fields or far away from a hospital, it gives you some indication of quite how well our bodies are designed for the job. Nature is a marvellous thing. When the brain perceives pain, with added stress, the body releases endorphins, a chemical compound with a pain-relieving effect **10 times more potent than morphine**. The more pain you have, the more endorphins that are released to help you cope.

As the endorphins build up you enter a state where your focus is internal rather than external. For some it is an almost dream-like state called 'labourland', for others it is one of intense awareness where you clock those around you with an intuitive sense of who they are and where they fit into the picture. The American midwife Kate Trishman, whom I met in the Taos Birth Centre, called this state being 'in the zone', describing the point when the labouring woman's rational thinking takes more of a backseat to her primitive being, when logical left-brain questions such as, 'Would you like ice chips with your glucose drink?' are near impossible to answer. You are, in one sense, away with the fairies.

Natural endorphins, as well as helping to push you into this primitive state, help you focus on what is happening inside you as opposed to what is going on outside. You may find yourself, as I did, connecting with only one or two people in the room who seemed crucial at that moment to birthing the baby – and in both my labours those people were midwives. The connection felt almost spiritual in its intensity, as if I were tapping into someone else's emotional reserves to help pull me through this experience and out through the other side. Mixed with the wonder of what is happening to your body, bringing forth a baby, it explains why many talk of a 'sacred energy' to the experience when it flows right.

Endorphins also help to colour your view of the birth afterwards, so that you recall it as an inner experience rather than an outer one, helping you to forget the pain (presumably so you go out and do it all over again a year or so later).

The Epidural Myth

By contrast, epidurals kill the natural endorphins and give you a completely different sort of experience. Once the needle is inserted into your back, the anaesthetic takes over the business of pain-relief and the natural endorphins are no longer needed in the body. Una, an acupuncturist who opted for an epidural in hospital when her labour didn't progress, described the sensation as being 'like having ice poured into your veins'. 'One moment I was aware of a discussion my husband and sister were having about who would be present when the baby was born, with me about to intervene gently. The next, after the epidural, I remember thinking "I don't fucking care."' With hindsight, Una wonders whether her sudden sense of detachment was caused not only by the epidural but also by the shock that accompanied the pain of the needle going into her back (in a case of rare bad luck, the anaesthetist took two attempts before inserting it correctly).

Without any wooziness from the endorphins, I remember my epidural birth as being hyper-real, an external rather than an internal experience, where the midwives holding my legs and the beeping monitors seemed to take centre-stage.

Epidurals still have a valuable place in modern obstetrics, particularly for 'back labours' when the baby is facing the wrong way round and labour progresses slowly, or for painful inductions when everything seems to be happening too fast. Then, they may be the answer to your prayers. But their reputation as solving the 'problem' of pain-relief is a myth. Epidurals come with a price. The bill may not have to be paid until after the birth, but your body will be the one forking out.

Life and Death

Jude Rachele made a spiritual connection on another level during her second birth with her twins. Her first son had been premature at 31 weeks, weighing only 3 lb 13 oz, and the birth came so unexpectedly that she 'did not have time to be truly conscious of the act, let alone attend antenatal classes'. Second time around, she was prepared for the twins to be early. Also, earlier in the year she had been through the death of her mother:

My first close death experience was courtesy of my mother who died from cancer. Her transition from life to death was one of the most beautiful, graceful, poetic experiences of my lifetime. I sat and watched. I learned. I listened. I did not fear the inevitable, and did my best through the depth of my love and compassion to usher my mother to her true resting point. She let go of her fear, she let go of her worry. She allowed herself to surrender to fate, the inevitability of her death, and basked in its warmth and glory.

It was then that I realized the labour of birth and the labour of death were virtually the same process. What remarkable experiences. And how blessed we are to be freely conscious beings at our deaths in a way we were not for the experience of our own births.

I took the power I derived from this experience into my next personal experience of birth. Just over one year after my mother's death I gave birth to my twin girls, and throughout my whole labour I visualized myself with my mother by her death bed. After my waters broke, I just lay quietly in my room by myself experiencing the contractions until my husband Rollin took me to hospital and I was checked as being 4 cm dilated. That was the first real indication that I accepted that my time had come. Now the real work was ahead of me.

With eyes closed and breath steady, I just sat back and remembered those last moments with the woman who loved me the most. I had been waiting for this opportunity for over two years, and was finally faced with one of the biggest challenges of my life. Birth can be so fearful, so painful and tense, but I refused to let my body and mind play tricks on me.

I had been very conscious of how important my mother's breathing was when we were told that she was dying, and we all sat around waiting for it to happen. I asked the medical staff in the hospital what I should be looking out for, and they said "her breathing". They told me that when she was close to death the breathing would become deeper and there would be more spaces between her breaths. My task was to keep my breath steady and not to let it get wildly out of control. Just stay calm, let your body do whatever it is it has to do, but just stay calm, and I re-experienced her last breaths.

In the room with me were my husband Rollin and a midwife, and at one point they began chit-chatting inanely over my belly, which began to break my concentration, so I had to ask them to be quiet and just to sit quietly in peace with me while this thing, labour, happened. They were pretty bored as I laboured, and I can remember the midwife commenting that in her 25 years as a midwife she had never seen anyone go through labour like this without pain-relief. She was astonished that I showed no outward expression or signs of being in labour, although I was wired up to monitors – in what felt like the most unnatural manner – which were ricocheting up and down as the contractions came and went. Sometime midway through my labour she asked if she could go get a cup of coffee and I could hear her sharing my tale in astonishment with the other midwives in the ward.

I existed with the peace and tranquillity of my own self-knowledge. When you learn to let go, even the pain of birth is a joy. Death is a joy. So many people fear death and spend a lifetime warding it off. Yet it is one of the most beautiful of life's experiences. I believe we need to stop clinging to the tangible and we need to start embracing the intangibles a lot more. In doing so, we can live a life without fear.

Jude went on to birth her first baby Amber without a hitch. Her second baby, Jasmine, was positioned with her arm next to her head, and the obstetrician decided to give Jude a spinal block in the operating theatre so that he could perform an internal version (move the baby into a better position). Jude rose to the challenge of remaining calm, relaxed and focused throughout, and Jasmine was born 1 hour and 7 minutes later, 'fearlessly, gracefully, thankfully'.

Don't Rush Me

While we are away with the fairies, I just wanted to say a short word about time. It doesn't really exist in the normal linear sense of the word when labouring. The idea of 'getting to work by 9 a.m.' when in labourland is as foreign as Korean Kim Chee soup. However, while you, the labouring woman, might not be aware of time, those around you will be.

Most hospitals have time-limits set for labour, based loosely on Friedman's Curve – a graph that plots cervical dilation [opening] against time in hours. However, a uterus, like most women, is extremely unpredictable, and has never been consistent at dilating at the standard 1cm an hour (a number that you should forget as soon as you have read it). Moreover, the time-limits were not invented to reassure women that the baby would come soon, but to have some sort of guide to process women through a maternity ward as quickly as possible. Friedman's Curve arrived in hospitals around the same time as 'active management' was introduced to a Dublin hospital and then rolled out across all hospitals in the UK.[1]

If labour is allowed to follow its natural course it is more likely to happen slower, not faster, than predicted. This is particularly true in hospital where the mother may be interrupted, given examinations, asked to lie on the bed and be monitored, and submit to other foreign ideas that don't concur with feeling relaxed and ready to give birth.

The American midwife Ina May Gaskin reports on one birth that shows how women can hold back from progressing for the most personal of reasons. After one labour was making good progress, the mother stopped dilating at 7cm and stuck there for a full day. In the process of exploring why labour might have stopped, the mother explained how, now the baby was coming, she regretted not making a lifetime commitment to her husband in her wedding vows a few months' earlier. In the interest of restarting labour, the midwife found someone to remarry the couple and include the phrase in the ceremony. Labour started again and the baby was born two hours later.

The reality of labour is that, as long as the mother and baby are being checked and deemed to be doing fine, labour can take as long or as short a time as the body and mind allow. There is no curve to follow, and labour can stop and start again for any number of reasons. **Labour often stops, for example, when a woman arrives in a maternity ward and the act of transferring her has caused the hormone adrenalin to kick in**, triggering 'fight or flight' mode, which inhibits labour. She may have been making good progress at home beforehand, but this alien environment has stopped all that until she feels comfortable again.

The long and short of it is that there is no long and short to it. If you and the baby are being monitored, and you are both in good nick, then there is no need to be rushed – even when you reach full dilation and you have no urge to push. 'Rest and be thankful' is what my midwife Mary Cronk used to repeat to me as she (patiently) saw in another dawn, day four, with me still waddling about the house contracting mildly.

Bach Flower Remedies

Bach Flower Remedies are a wonderful way of fine-tuning our psychospiritual selves. If you know anything about Bach Flower Remedies it will probably be because of that little yellow bottle of Rescue Remedy that is now so ubiquitous that it is even sold in Boots. It is there to treat shock, and if you haven't yet added one to your medicine chest, then now is the time to do so. Like homoeopathic Arnica, flower remedies are harmless to children and can even be used, with advice, on babies. I'm currently giving a mixture made by a homoeopath to my three-year-old daughter to help with her night tantrums. 'Mummy, can I have my fairy medicine now?' she asks every evening after her bath.

What is useful about Bach Flower Remedies is the process of self-discovery that accompanies a diagnosis. If you are lucky enough to be introduced to the remedies by a Bach Flower practitioner (usually found wherever homoeopathy is practised), then they may recommend a special formula to help you during the run-up to the birth. The practitioner will explore your feelings around the birth, and perhaps diagnose something like Star of Bethlehem for a previous trauma, or Mimulus if you are nervous.

Alternatively, you can buy a book and diagnose yourself. In the later stages of my pregnancy I spent a lot of time floating around in the bath reading my Bach Flower Remedy book. When I went overdue I would put a few drops of Walnut in the bath, having read 'A person in the Walnut state finds it hard to take that final step, some negative aspects of her personality still being caught up, consciously or unconsciously, in old decisions and bonds from the past.' 'Oh, yes,' I'd think, 'that's a bit of me. I need help with "my new beginnings in a mental and spiritual sphere". I think I'll whack in a few more drops.' Then I'd read on and come to Impatiens: 'Impatiens relates to the soul qualities of patience and gentleness. In the negative Impatiens state we are impatient, inner tension tending to make us irritable towards others.' 'Oh yes, that's also me, I shouldn't have snapped at Adam today, so I'll add another few drops of that to the hot water, too.' I also made a pipette bottle up to swig at during labour, with Evian water and a few drops of Rescue Remedy.

Like homoeopathy, if you don't diagnose yourself correctly with a Flower remedy, no harm will be done. 'If a flower frequency is not the right one, the Higher Self recognizes it as such and it is not admitted to our energetic system. It will have no effect, therefore, unlike medicaments given in material doses which will always have an effect on the metabolism,' writes Mechthild Scheffer in her book *Bach Flower Therapy: Theory and Practice* (HarperCollins, 1998).

Bach Flower Remedies can be bought in any good health food shop or, along with the bottles to make up a swigging potion, from The Organic Pharmacy at just under £4 per remedy at the time of writing (tel.: 0207 351 2232; www.theorganicpharmacy.com). If you have a Yorkshireman reading over your shoulder and shaking his head at this moment, settle for a bottle of Rescue Remedy from Boots for the big day, and let your birth assistant swig away, too.

For God's Sake, Give Me Some Proper Drugs

Remember, there are no medals for giving birth without pain-relief. It is seen as a desirable goal because it helps you to feel in control of what is happening and shortens the recovery period afterwards. It also makes you tremendously pleased and proud of yourself, as if you just passed your driving test and won the Nobel Peace Prize on the same day. If, however, being 'in control' includes ingesting whatever drugs the medical

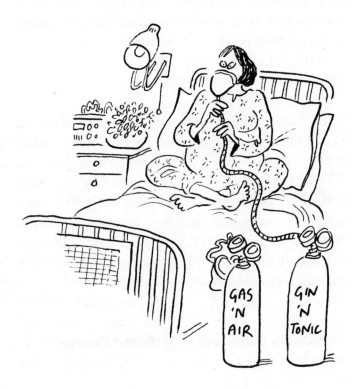

establishment might offer, here is what they currently dole out if you shout loudly enough. Just don't confuse pain-relief with anaesthesia. Pain-relief helps you to manage your own pain, anaesthesia takes away your control.

TENS MACHINE

This never worked for me; I found it was like having an annoying transistor radio attached to my side. However, many women swear by it in early labour and can use it successfully at home on their own. The machine works by deflecting the body's attention away from the pain of a contraction by issuing electronic impulses which can be increased manually, like turning up the volume on a stereo, as the contraction increases. The concept is rather like digging your nails into the palm of your hand to distract you from the pain elsewhere. They can be hired from Boots and other chemists, and have the advantage of being tried out ahead of time. Mine was ripped off early on, to be followed by a plea for something more hardcore.

ENTONOX - GAS AND AIR

This involves sucking on a tube, or through a mouth-piece, to take the edge off a contraction. It definitely makes you a little high, which is an advantage or disadvantage depending on what floats your boat. Some, like me, love it, others, like my friend Rikke, didn't. She likened it to smoking marijuana (which is not advisable as a form of relaxation when labour starts, as one girl-friend found out to her cost while lying paranoid in the bath). The technique with gas and air is to start sucking on the mouthpiece as soon as you feel the contraction starting, so that at the peak of the contraction you have taken in enough of the stuff to ride the wave. It has no after-effects – the feeling-woozy sensation goes away immediately. Gas and air is available for home births.

EPIDURAL OR SPINAL BLOCK

This is anaesthesia administered through a needle in the spine to numb you from the waist downwards. Although it may be offered routinely, it is a form of intervention and, like all interventions, may result in additional measures such as an IV drip to strengthen contractions, constant electronic foetal monitoring, forceps or a ventouse, to birth the baby. However, there are occasions when it is particularly useful, such as for 'back' labours, when the baby's spine is opposite your own and labour is that much more difficult and painful (see Epidural Birth, page 183).

This was the case for my firstborn, and after a long labour that wasn't progressing the epidural allowed me to relax and progress from 5 cm dilation to 10 cm (Bingo) in 20 minutes. The baby's position gave me bad backache and I had 'frozen' at 5 cm. Although, as already described, the experience was very different from the ecstatic birth of the twins, the epidural never the less served an efficient medical purpose. One after-effect was a nagging backache where the needle was inserted. Not everyone has this, but I did.

PETHIDINE

This is a morphine derivative which can be used for home births along with gas and air (for obvious reasons, an epidural needs a skilled anaesthetist and thus is only available in hospital). Pethidine is a synthetic narcotic, an analgesic (pain-relieving) drug usually admitted by intramuscular injection that works powerfully within 20 minutes and lasts between two and four hours, depending on the size of the dose. It is not an anaes-thetic but a muscle-relaxant and mood-enhancer, affecting your perception of the pain, and is usually given with an antihistamine to counteract any feelings of nausea. It is not so popular these days because the drug crosses the placenta and can make the baby drowsy if delivery follows soon after the drug is admin-istered. Despite this, my midwife Mary Cronk says that her notes from 20 years ago showed comparatively large doses of pethidine given to mothers during labour, with good outcomes for the mothers and babies.

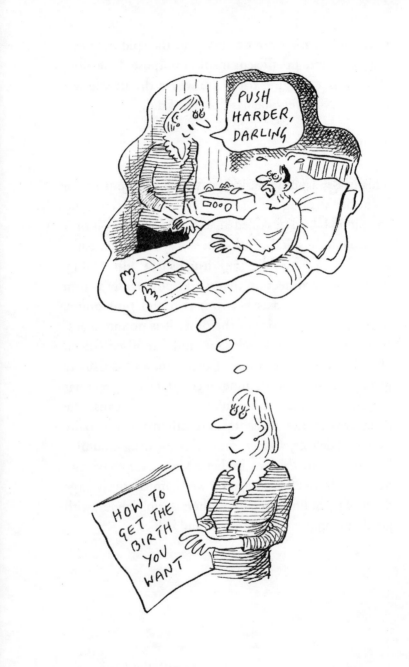

SECOND STAGE

BIRTH STORIES:
BRILLIANT WAYS
TO GIVE BIRTH

7

Introduction: Water, Water Everywhere

As you are about to find out, water plays a big part during many women's labours – whether they are taking a shower, contracting away happily in the bath, or deciding not to get into a birth pool because they want their feet on *terra firma* (with husband totting up in his head how much the pool cost to hire). Either way, water is one of the easiest ways to relax during labour. Freed from gravity's pull, the lack of stress allows the endorphin levels to climb and the mother to focus inwardly on the birth process. Aaaahhhhhh.

Not that we are the first generation to know this. An old book called *Water Cures*, printed in London in 1723, described the benefit of bathing during labour. Even further back, the ancient Egyptians birthed selected babies, chosen to be future priests and priestesses, under water. Normal fears of babies drowning vanish when mothers learn that their infants continue to take in oxygen through the umbilical cord until they make contact with the air. One friend, Caddy, who had a wonderful water birth for her second child, held him gently at the water's surface before asking the midwife when he would start breathing. 'Blow gently on his eyelids,' replied the midwife, and Caddy did, watching his eyes flutter open and her baby take his very first breath.

Birthing in water has lots of benefits for the baby. 'During the birth, babies often open their eyes, move in all directions, and use their limbs. Water mitigates the shock and sensory overload that are often an inextricable part of birth' writes Barbara Harper, herself a veteran water-birther and author of *Gentle Birth Choices* (Healing Arts Press, 1997).

The French physician Michel Odent, former head of surgery at a state hospital in Pithiviers in France, has done more to introduce the benefits of water birth to the modern woman than any other man alive. In his book *Birth Reborn*, Odent comments: 'Some women who are strongly drawn to water throughout pregnancy are even more attracted to it during labour. Still others tell us that they don't like the water or can't swim. Yet as labour begins, these same women will suddenly move toward the pool, enter eagerly and not want to leave.' Some women feel the urge to leave the pool just before birth (see Emma King's story, page 119). Some experience what Odent calls 'the fetal ejection reflex' when they enter the cooler temperature of the air and the change of environment triggers an adrenalin release, and the baby is born in one contraction (see Janet Balaskas' story, page 195 – she was attended by Odent for her third birth).

On the occasion of his 100th water birth, Odent published an article in *The Lancet* relating his views on water birth:

We have found no risk attached either to labour or to birth underwater. The use of warm water during labour requires further research, but we hope that other experience would confirm that immersion in warm water is an efficient, easy and economical way to reduce the use of drugs and the rate of intervention in parturition.[1]

More recently further research has been carried out. In January 2004 the *British Medical Journal* published findings online from a study of 99 women. The University of Southampton showed that women who spent at least part of their labour in water had less pain, and were less likely to need an epidural or require induction to speed up their contractions than those cared for in the conventional way. Overall, women who used the pool felt more satisfied with the way the birth had gone. These findings are important to encourage maternity units, more than 90 per cent of which have birthing pools and baths, to open their doors a little wider. Britain is currently the leader worldwide in offering water birth facilities, and yet only 2 per cent of women in hospitals use them.[2] Common safety fears from medical professionals include: the inability to use an electronic foetal monitor on the mother while she is in water, the need to keep everything sterile (ordinary tap water is used with no harmful effects for mother or baby) and, if the pools are deep, how the midwife can have proper access to the mother.

In the following stories, none of the three mothers who birthed their babies at home, in hospital and in a birth centre was troubled by these fears as they stuck their toes in the water, and all were attended by midwives who were experienced in the medium. Like all the birth stories recounted in the following pages, **they are personal and positive experiences, so you have nothing to fear from reading them**.

All the birth stories are told in the mothers' own words [with square brackets like these from me when I can't resist interrupting with information or explanation] and they cover the whole range of experiences from aquatic to Caesarean section. Their aim is to demystify birth to the uninitiated or offer a different approach for those who have been there, done that and worn the bloody T-shirt. Enjoy.

8

Water Birth in Hospital

When Emma King, 36, gave birth to her first child, Charlie, in Queen Charlotte's Hospital in West London, it was the hottest day of the year. She had attended NCT classes and enlisted the help of a male midwife on the one-to-one scheme, and had an empowering, drug-free labour.

Right at the beginning of the pregnancy, at the 12 week scan, I wanted to get on to the one-to-one midwife scheme [where you have continuity of care throughout pregnancy and birth] because we lived 5 minutes from Queen Charlotte's Hospital in Hammersmith, West London. The scheme was being expanded in the area, and at my first meeting with the doctor he asked whether I'd mind having a male midwife. I said 'No' without giving it much thought. I think there were quite a few women who didn't want a man, and there were a couple of times during the pregnancy when I met him and thought, 'Help. I don't want a man at the birth! I want a woman who has preferably had a baby already. What does he know, he's only a man!' But my midwife Sudess was terribly laid-back about everything, which was perfect for me.

At the first meeting I thought he would take charge, and he didn't. He kind of let me take charge, and I tried to lay the law down, about how I wanted an epidural as soon as the first contraction came, and how I wanted to take drugs and I just didn't want to have the pain, and he just nodded sagely and let me rant. And, in retrospect, I know he was thinking 'Here's a challenge.' Or 'Let's just see how she changes her mind during her pregnancy.' A real plus to the one-to-one scheme was that I didn't have to go to hospital except for the two scans during my whole pregnancy.

He came to the house and got to know me a bit, and I felt like a name, not a number. I didn't stop working until a month before the birth, but I had done NCT classes. The NCT classes were good for me because I met other mothers in the same predicament, and they were all first-timers, too. The NCT woman wasn't exactly inspiring, however. She had about 18 children herself, and looked pale, thin, wan and really, really tired. I remember laughing with another girl there about how she wasn't a good advert for motherhood.

The turning-point on the NCT course was when the teacher fell ill and we had the independent midwife Caroline Flint [former head of the Royal College of Midwives who now runs her own private birth centre in south London]. Caroline demonstrated everything, and was completely gung-ho about acting it out, she was doing a mock imitation of a woman in labour pacing around the room going 'Oh my God!' and that made it really real. It was animated for the first time. Caroline made a big click for me, because it was the first time I thought about natural birth – without painkillers and epidural – that it could be a viable option. I think because, through her demonstration, it seemed copable with, it wasn't such a mystery.

Caroline was also very strident about how your birth should be how you want it to be. She was very forthright about that, and that you had every right to have it how you wanted (at which point she gave out leaflets about her birth centre), for a few thousand pounds! But she was pointing out that you had a choice, and she also made the whole drug options sound awful.

She painted the drugs as 'if you needed it, there was nothing wrong with you needing it' – she didn't come down on it in an awful negative way, like the thin, pale, wan other teacher had. She told the story of helping her own daughter give birth and giving her pethidine when she wanted it, so it wasn't like this complete taboo. But she did come up with all these statistics saying recovery was better, it was better for the baby – the drugs didn't cross the placenta – and all that stuff. And that was a bit of a turning-point for me, and she talked about doing a birth plan. I had read about birth plans, but not done one, so the next time I saw Sudess, I had done my birth plan [see Third Stage – Eight Weeks to Go, page 242 for suggested birth plans].

My birth plan said that I wanted to be in a pool, although I wrote that I didn't want to give birth in it. I knew that Queen Charlotte's had the option of a pool, Sudess had told me, and also he said that he had done a lot of water births and the one-to-one midwives were very pro water births (although the regular hospital midwives didn't seem to be). Sudess said that every water birth that he had ever done had been really fantastic for everybody there. And he didn't push me, but he encouraged me to think about it. And it did cost at Queen Charlotte's — it's free at Hammersmith's for example — but at Charlotte's you had to book the bath, and it was about £150 for the liner to line the bath. So I booked that, and put it in the birth plan.

I went into labour five days before my due date. On the Saturday we'd had a lovely day and gone for a picnic, had dinner with friends at their house. During dinner this girl really made me laugh and I remember feeling a little 'pop'. Then I went to the loo and was sitting on the loo for hours thinking, 'This is the longest pee I've ever done in my life' — it was my waters breaking. Then I went downstairs and thought, 'I've got to get home,' and [husband] Stuart had drunk a bottle of red wine so I realized that I had to drive.

I rang Sudess, got his answerphone, and his partner Lesley came round instead. She did a stick test on the fluid to check whether it was amniotic, and it was. She said, 'I can't stay because I've got to get to hospital, I've got another woman who's contracting like a train.'

So we went to bed, and the fluid trickled to nothing. The following day, Sudess called me around 10 a.m. and said that technically I should come into hospital 24 hours after my waters had broken if labour hadn't started. 'But seeing as your waters broke at midnight, why don't you come in at 8 p.m. and we'll check you then,' he suggested. So we had a normal Sunday, I remember twinges but nothing that wasn't a Braxton Hicks, and we went in at 8 p.m. to be checked for dilation and to be given a 'sweep' [a midwife's gloved finger run around the rim of the cervix] to get things going. And I remember reading my notes later, and seeing that at that point I was 2-3 cm dilated, and I'm really grateful that he didn't make me stay in the hospital. He was very pro-home birth and for being at home for as long as possible, as he said in his experience labour progresses much better that way.

He said, 'I think you should come back in at 7 a.m.,' and he was very categorical about the time, 7 a.m., it was a time engraved in my brain. So we went home and went to bed, again. After about 20 minutes in bed, it was now about 11 o'clock, and the contractions were beginning to kick in, so I got up and watched a bit of telly and spent the night padding around the flat on my own. I was really grateful to be on my own, and glad it was night, I didn't want Stuart there, I liked privately monitoring my own body. I was messing about with the TENS machine for hours, trying to get it to work and seeing whether it made any difference – that was a very good distraction.

By about 2 a.m. the contractions started to get a bit heavy, and I went to every room in the flat trying to find a comfortable position to be in, with Caroline Flint coming back into my head at that point. I curled up on the spare bed with about 100 cushions for a while, then I leaned on the kitchen sideboard. All the time, in my head, I was thinking 'If I can get to 7 o'clock, it'll all be fine.' I was thinking, 'I can't ring Sudess before that time, he needs his sleep,' and it was a bit like not waking up Stuart because I thought: why should they be woken up when they can't really do anything? Just before 6 a.m., I was hyper-aware of my body, in the way that you are, and I was thinking about it going OK and thinking, 'I'm on the run now, and this is the moment I've waited for all my life, labour and its ghastliness, and now I'm going through it.'

By 6 a.m. I thought, 'I want to go to hospital and have an epidural, it's too tiring, and it hurts too much.' I waited until 6.15 a.m. and then I called Sudess. I mentioned the epidural when I spoke to him and he sort of brushed over it, saying, 'OK, whatever' in a way that suggested that I'd forget about it by the time I got to the hospital. He said 'When are the contractions coming?' and I said 'I don't know, but there's not that much time between them.' At 10 to 7 I took Stuart a cup of tea and said, 'I think we should go to the hospital.'

Sudess was where he said he'd be, and said, 'How are you?' and I said, 'In labour!' I lay on the bed and he checked my dilation: I was 7-8 cm at that stage, but he didn't tell me that, he said, 'Oh, you're about 7,' and he admitted later that I was nearer 8 but he didn't want to tell me, because he didn't want it to slow up. Every bit of information that he gave me, he gave me slightly less than the reality, which was good because it made me feel better when I got on to the next level before I was expecting to.

The pool thing took ages, because the liner had to be put in and then the pool had to be filled (and I was expecting that the pool would be ready for me to get into). So Stuart and Sudess were DIY men with this birth pool, and I was every now and then clutching the side, saying 'Could you get on with it?' Filling the pool took over an hour. I was wearing a dress which was all I wore for the last month of pregnancy, and I didn't really want the dress on, but I didn't want it off either while they were filling up the pool. And then they were taking the temperature and faffing about, and then I had to get into the pool, finding the moment to swing my leg over between contractions. Suddenly stripping off was strange, because Sudess had never seen me naked, he'd never seen anything of me except when I first went in and he gave me a sweep. But at that point I didn't really care.

Getting in the pool was heaven. It was warm, it was all-surrounding, I could blob about a bit, and didn't have this full weight, and it was just the next stage. It was the equivalent of being really hot and getting into a swimming pool – instant relief. The contractions kept on going, and every now and then Sudess would lean over the side and check me for dilation.

After about an hour and a half, he said 'You might get an urge to push, and if you do, that's fine.' And it was almost like power of suggestion – 5 minutes later I did get an urge to push. It was like he pre-empted everything, so there was never a shock element. When I got the urge to push, I also got the urge to get out of the pool. I think I did one push and then I wanted to get out. So I got onto the bed and was kneeling, holding onto the back of the bed, and he said, 'When you feel the urge to push, just push.' I was having some lower back pain, and he alleviated that by pushing really hard on my lower back, and showed Stuart how to do the same. He was also helping with the breathing.

The pushing went on for ages, it went on for over an hour. I had the fan that we had brought in, blowing away on me. Stuart was dripping with sweat, he said afterwards that he was so hot that he thought he was going to explode. After an hour, Sudess told us that he was going to have to tell the registrar that I had been pushing for over an hour, because of hospital rules. At that point my heart sank, because I thought 'Oh no, it's going to be a ventouse, or intervention of some sort, and I've come this far …' So he went off to tell the doctor, having monitored me and found out that the baby was OK.

Then, the Head Consultant of Charlotte's came in with some other people, and I was bellowing like a cow. She came right up to me, put her hand on my arm and said, 'You must be quite tired because you've been pushing a long time' and I said, 'I am.' And she said, 'When the next contraction comes, concentrate as much as you can on the contraction and try and channel the sound you are making into the push.' So don't make the sound, put it into the push. I knew it had gone onto a different level even though Sudess was there, because 'doctors' were in the room. It was such good advice, because I pushed, and I only needed two or three pushes with her there and the head came out (I later found out that Charlie had his hand by his head, so he got stuck when turning, and that was what was slowing things up). Stuart was up by my head supporting me at that stage, and I was aware that I didn't want him down the other end either.

When the head was out, I was told to give one more push for the shoulders. So Charlie came out, Sudess caught him, and how great was that! The baby cried, and Stuart cried, and I was just so relieved it was all over. [Stuart says: 'I was just trying to imagine what Emma was feeling as she was going through it. There's never another point where you feel more drawn together through one act. There's not even a comparison to when you are beginning to make the baby. And when the baby's head starts to come out, you've been living with this for nine months and then finally you think "My God', he's really here."']

Then, as quickly as the entourage came in, they left. A student had already come in earlier in the pushing stage and asked whether she could have the placenta for some research purposes, and I shouted 'Yes, yes, whatever ... let's get the baby out first.' But I had forgotten that you have to push the placenta out. I hadn't read that chapter in the book. I was still on my hands and knees, and Sudess said, 'You have to push out the placenta' and I said 'I can't.' And he said, 'You can, and you will, and you actually have to.' And I was like, 'Oh how long will it take?' I remember being amazed at the amount of blood everywhere, and thinking 'I'm glad I didn't have it at home.'

I did have the injection [syntocinon to help expel the placenta] although I had put on my birth plan that I didn't want it unless I needed it. But because the pushing had gone on for so long, they wanted to wrap things up. And Sudess could have said at that point, 'We're going to hang, draw and quarter you' and I would have said, 'Oh OK, because you are my hero and I'll do whatever you say.' He played me really well, and I didn't give him credit for that in the beginning. He probably recognized that I was a total control freak, but he gave me enough information to go on, and I trusted him. And it was so great to know that he was going to be there all the time; I don't know what I'd have done if we'd suddenly changed midwives in a shift, which happens to so many other people.

So then I was turned round to give Charlie a feed, and he breastfed immediately. I felt on a different planet, I felt so proud and suddenly it was like 'Here is the baby.' It's like climbing a mountain and seeing a marvellous view, and you can't quite believe that you've made it to the top. And I had done it without drugs, and that was a really big thing for me. Because I never thought I'd be one of those people who could. Then we had photos of Charlie being weighed, and Charlie was very alert, his apgar scores [see page 251] were 9 and 10, and he looked very sweet because he had all this hair, like a mini punk. Sudess then left us alone for about an hour in the delivery room, and we had a lovely time, all gooey moments, until a wheelchair appeared and we were to be wheeled down to the ward to stay in overnight. I remember thinking 'But I'm fine. I can walk.'

9

Water Birth at Home

Sasha and Dominic Dromgoole have three daughters, all born normally – two in hospital and one at home. Husband Dominic was a keen participant in all of Sasha's births, defending and supporting her decision to birth where she wanted, and bonding instantly with his daughters, he feels, by being involved. For Sasha's second birth at home, described below, Dominic stuck his head into the pool to watch his daughter appear. 'It was incredibly peaceful with no sense of hurry,' he describes. 'I saw this head coming down, and I watched as she opened her eyes and turned looking from side to side, noticeably calm. Even now she is the most calm in the family, I think largely because of her birth.' Sasha, 28 at the time of Grainne's birth, picks up the story after her first daughter's birth.

After Siofra's birth in hospital, I felt exhilarated by the experience but knew that I didn't really want to go into hospital again for the second baby. I had done some yoga classes and wanted to be in control, and I was lucky that they had a one-to-one scheme in the area [as in Emma's story, page 119, this is where the NHS offer continuity of care with the same mid-wife through pregnancy and birth]. When I told my midwife Jean Reid that I was thinking about a home birth, she was enthusiastic, saying, 'Home births are wonderful, if this is what you want, let's go for it.' She was always positive. It was just an inkling of an idea, but Jean encouraged and made it possible, and Dom was up for an adventure.

I'd heard other women come in during my pregnancy yoga class and give their birth stories, and the home birth stories seemed happier: the women always said, 'It was wonderful for the babies and they were much calmer.' Siofra had had a lot of colic from 6 p.m. to 9 p.m. every day, and was very clingy and difficult, and I think that came from a difficult start in life.

For this baby I wanted to try for an easy birth, I feel that birth is the first informative experience for the baby, and I believe if it's happy and good then that's going to feed into her per-manently. They are born into their characters. Homoeopaths always ask about the birth, as if it has an influence on the child's personality and physiognomy. ['I loved watching all of my daughters being born, it's so connected with their per-sonality and who they are,' adds Dominic.]

I also wanted Siofra to be involved. She was only 18 months old, and I didn't want to be away from her while in hospital. I decided that if Siofra was awake she could be there, and we all watched videos together of natural births and water births to prepare her. I made everyone who was around watch them – even the German *au pair*. [Dominic adds: 'Everyone was delighted to watch it, although I am suspicious of the psychology of the people who where in it, they were fairly Hippy Dippy, and it was a little bit forced and "aren't we perfect?"']

It felt like a revelation, we didn't have to go to hospital at all after the five-month scan. Towards the end, Jean would come over twice a week, we'd have a cup of tea and a laugh for half an hour, and sometimes if it was lunchtime she'd sit and have lunch with us. She was always very respectful of the fact that it was our house and made friends with Siofra, so she was like part of the family. She'd feel the shape of the baby and that felt very intimate and quite physical. She kept all the stuff needed for the birth in a drawer in the kitchen and we ordered the birth pool two weeks before it was needed.

But Grainne's due date came and went. If she went overdue by two weeks, Jean said she would have to be induced, which would mean a hospital birth. So, 10 days' overdue, we decided we would try and kickstart things and she would give me a sweep at home [when the midwife puts her fingers in to feel the cervix, a procedure that can sometimes induce labour]. Meanwhile I drank gallons of raspberry-leaf tea and massaged clary sage oil into my ankles. The night before Jean was due to give the sweep we had a huge curry and my brother brought some marijuana over. I'd heard smoking grass could work, and by this time was ready to try anything. We got wonderfully stoned and laughed and laughed, and by the time I got to bed I thought I could feel something happening. I laboured very gently through the night, sleeping through it mostly. When Jean came for the sweep at 11 a.m. I was already 3 cm dilated.

She said, 'We're OK, you might even have it today.' Dom was told not to go to work, and instead took an enormous pile of sheets round to the laundrette. I gave Siofra her lunch, which calmed me as the contractions grew stronger, and then the *au pair* Michelle took her off to the park. So I was alone when my forewaters broke and the contractions suddenly set in hard and strong, so that I had to work through them. I went up to the bathroom, stood in the empty bath and laboured there waiting, mildly panicked that no one was there. But they all turned up a moment later. My waters were clear and beautiful, silvery like silicon, and they were like a splash of light, making my legs shiny. The time was around 11.45 a.m.

Dom and Jean turned up at about the same time and everything kicked off. Jean massaged my lower back while I groaned away, standing and rotating my hips in the bathroom, and occasionally popped downstairs to check on the progress of the water pool that was being filled. At some point I became absolutely desperate to get into the water. The contractions were coming faster and harder and I wanted some kind of relief. But the water in the birthing pool had to be at a certain temperature before I could get in, and we had just run out of hot water. While we were waiting for the water to reheat, Dom went to the neighbours either side for pans and kettles in a Blitz effort to get water into the pool.

Eventually there was sufficient hot water to cover me if I lay on my side, and I came down with Jean around 1 o'clock to get into the pool.

As soon as I got into the pool, I relaxed. It was wonderful. I submerged myself completely, I wanted to be right under the water. I breathed out through the contractions, completely submerged, and then came up for breath. Everyone was busying themselves around me, but I felt safe because I was at home. Siofra was tired when she came back from the park and waved at me as she was falling asleep in Michelle's arms being taken upstairs (that was a relief, because the last thing I wanted was to look after her at that moment). But the fact that she waved and was happy made it lovely to have her in the house.

At that moment, Jean said 'Dom should be with you now, I'll take over for a bit,' and I asked Dom to hold my head as I got into a meditative breath. The contractions were like a hurricane going on around me, and I was in the eye of the storm. It felt as if the pain was happening around me but I'd found a safe place at the centre of it, it was really weird. I was right inside it. The contractions were coming in waves and there was no space between them now, just one after the other rolling over me. I didn't feel the pain. I was so peaceful, I was so relaxed, and the fact that the midwife was even thinking about and looking after Dom meant that I could relax and visualize what was happening, with Dom holding my head and the 'waves' going over me.

I remember hearing snatches of conversation as people were just getting on with their business. I felt supported but not stared at or stood over.

When I went into transition [the period between first and second stage of pushing in labour], I suddenly wanted to get out of the bath and was feeling a little sick. There was an odd pause for about 15 minutes in which I began to wonder if anything would happen at all. Then the pushing contractions came. Suddenly I didn't want to be in the water anymore. I stood up in the water and wanted to push. Jean didn't check that I was fully dilated but said, 'If you want to push, have a go.' I did, and as I did my coccyx clicked up and I thought, 'This isn't right.' This was the only time I panicked in the whole birth, and I even saw a trace of anxiety on Jean's face (she later told me that big babies have occasionally been known to damage their mother's back, and Grainne turned out to be 10 lb and I'm only 5 ft 3 inches, and quite small), but she remained completely calm at the time. I was worried because my brother had broken his back, and I thought, 'I can't push or it might happen to me.' Jean said, 'Don't push, just lay down and relax.'

I lay down in the pool again and Jean said, 'Your baby is there, I've felt the head. Put your hand down and feel the baby's head.' I put my hand between my legs and I could feel her hair, her soft pulpy head and, as I felt it, a wave of relaxation went through me. Suddenly everything made sense: the shape of her, the shape of me, what we were trying to achieve together. Jean told me not to push but just to 'breathe the baby out' with the contractions. At the next contraction and breath, the contraction was doing it, I was lying on my side and the contraction pushed her head out first with my hand still over her head, and then her arms. 'Your baby's there, it's reaching up for you, look,' said Jean. I looked down and these two little arms reached up towards me. 'Take her,' said Jean. So I put my hands under her armpits and pushed, and gently pulled with the next contraction and she seemed to wriggle her way out, helping me. Dominic was supporting my leg and I pulled her gently out, so that she floated up to the surface with me holding her. When she was at the surface she naturally breathed. Her eyes were wide open and she seemed to see us all. She looked around the room and it really felt as if she had just swum into the world.

She was so peaceful. It felt as if she knew the house and all the voices around her, which of course she did. Then the family turned up en masse and we had a fish and chips feast. Grainne was wrapped up and put to one side, sleeping really happily, while we sat down to eat it. It was all very calm.

10

Laughter Birth

Whenever Linsey McNeill watched a drama on television, with a woman screaming while giving birth, her mother used to tut and say 'It's not like that in real life, you know, it's much calmer.' As Linsey approached the birth of her first child, she wrote a birth plan asking for all the drugs listed. 'I thought, "why go through any pain?" So when I was in labour and into my routine, it was painful, but it was just like Mum said it would be – a positive pain, and I wanted to stay with the pain because I knew what was happening and going on. And I really enjoyed it, knowing that my body could take that level of pain and I was in control of it. It was the first time I felt I was really totally in control of anything.' Linsey also managed to see the funny side of giving birth, with the help of a strange hand movement and the odd giggle.

My pregnancy was hideous right through: I had terrible morning sickness and I found the whole thing very stressful. At five weeks I started to bleed and I bled all the way through the pregnancy. At the scans they were worried that the baby was too small, and kept asking me in for more appointments, and my overall feeling was that pregnancy was an illness. On top of it all we moved house when I was 7 months' pregnant, and the new house was a wreck that we were doing up.

At 35 weeks the new house was so disgusting that I thought 'I'm driving up to Mum's.' I drove from London to Sheffield and Mum wasn't there, she'd gone shopping. So I walked in through her door, which seemed an oasis of calm and cleanliness after what I'd left behind, and as I stepped over the threshold my waters broke. I was pretty sure that I was in labour. I called my sister-in-law, who was a midwife, and she said, 'It definitely sounds like labour, get yourself to hospital.'

My brother drove me to the Jessop Hospital in Sheffield, insisting that I sit on his laminated street map to prevent any damage to his car seat! I wasn't booked in there but I did have my hand-held notes with me. The doctor came to see me and did the litmus test to check whether the water was amniotic fluid and said, 'No, you've got a weak bladder,' which both my brother and I found hilarious. So I went back home to Mum's at about 5 p.m. and then started getting labour pains and contractions around midnight. I went back into hospital, and the same doctor came and apologized, saying 'Sorry you *were* in labour, we made a mistake.' They checked me and I was 5 cm dilated.

I thought, 'Big problem. I'm here but [my husband] Tom's not,' and he definitely wanted to be there – he'd catalogued the whole labour from the baby being the size of a strawberry. I thought, 'I've got to get him here.' It was 2 a.m. and I was in hospital with my mum and sister. He managed to get on the first train at 9 a.m. Mum was really panicking, but for the first time during my pregnancy I felt really calm. I felt comfortable that I was in the right place, even though I wasn't, I was 170 miles away from home. Because it was my home town and everyone talked like me it felt right. I hated the hospital in London and none of that had mattered at all except when I was in labour. I loved the fact that in the Jessop the cleaning lady sounded like my grandmother. It just felt so right.

The doctor came to see me and said, 'We can put you in an ambulance and send you back down to London,' because I seemed to have stopped dilating at 5 cm. Tom had just arrived and I thought, 'I'm not shifting, I want to have the baby here.' She said, 'Well, we're going to induce you, then' to speed up the contractions. Tom went back to my brother's flat for a rest while they set me up with a drip to induce me.

I was sitting on the bed reading *Marie Claire* and my Mum popped in. I'd been feeling absolutely fine, but the moment Mum came in through the door I had the first enormous contraction. I was panicking, thinking 'What's happening?' and Mum said 'Stay calm, breathe, think of it like the ocean, you're pushing back the ocean with your breath.'

So I lay back, closed my eyes and I started doing this hand movement [the hand movement was made up on the spot and consisted of a beckoning gesture followed by a pushing-away motion]. I could feel the contractions but I just didn't care. I was almost in a trance, and I felt completely connected to the baby, and was really happy, really pleased to be there. And I wasn't thinking, 'Soon I'm going to have a baby.' I was thinking, 'Soon I'm going to stop feeling so sick.'

Every so often I would giggle at the thought of how ridiculous I must look 'doing the locomotion' with my hands, eyes closed. There was a junior doctor with me and I knew she was thinking 'What's she's doing? She's probably some sort of new-age lunatic hippie,' but she just held my other hand, and as long as she didn't speak and just held my hand that was fine. If anyone came and tried to interrupt me, I found it was an intrusion. I just wanted to stay in my own little world, I didn't want anyone in my world with me. I just wanted to be there on my own. My mum kept putting cold cloths on my head, and I didn't even know that I wanted them but they were just perfect. I was hot and they kept me cool and calm.

After two hours of 'pushing back the waves', a doctor came in. He said, 'You're going to be like this for another 10 hours' – but instead of feeling deflated, I thought 'Fine I can cope, I can do this.' Just after he left, I felt this enormous pain, which I didn't know at the time but was the head engaging. I went into a panic again – the contractions had been painful, but this pain was so bad that that I said to Mum 'Could you get me an epidural?' But I knew even as I said it that I couldn't stay still for them to put in a needle and I suddenly got the giggles again, thinking 'What am I going to do now?' I also found it funny that here I was strapped up in this position, and I was the one who had got myself into this mess. For some reason, all of this struck me at the time as hilarious.

My nice midwife and doctor had gone out for a cup of tea, and a new midwife came in, and I announced 'I'm going to have the baby soon,' and she said 'No, you're not!' Then she lifted up the sheet and looked, turned to my mum and said: 'Get the father!'

Mum came back in and said 'I can't get hold of Tom, the phone's engaged, you'll just have to do it without him.' And I said, 'No way! You'll just have to get in your car, drive there and bring him back.' The nice midwife said 'OK, we can wait. Take some gas and air and we'll wait.' I knew Tom would be devastated if I gave birth without him.

At one stage, the midwife said 'I've lost the baby's heartbeat; you're going to have to start pushing,' but I knew the belt had just slipped and everything was OK, and I thought 'No, I'm not giving birth without Tom here.' And I knew that he couldn't be too far away.

I felt really calm. I felt like I wanted to go into a cave and be all alone in the wilderness. I felt connected with the baby and I felt everything was connected. I felt connected to Mum because I thought this is what she went through when she had me, and I felt that it was me and the baby going through the labour.

After a couple of pathetic pushes (I wasn't really trying), Tom came bowling in and the midwife said 'We've got the father – let's push!' At that stage I was holding on to Mum's arm and I needed her to prop me up. I had Tom on one side, my Mum on the other, and with one push Emelye was out – she almost arrived with Tom. And she was absolutely fine. The crash team were on standby with the special care unit, but she was fine – as I knew all along she would be.

Everything went really well, and I remember thinking the whole experience was really enjoyable and really funny, from my waters breaking and my bladder being considered too weak onwards. Despite everyone panicking around me, I was calm. I think it showed that doctors can't know everything and sometimes you have to rely on your own instincts. Emelye was 5 lb 1 oz, and she stayed in special care for a week until she developed a sucking reflex.

I was amazed that I could do it. I faint at the sight of blood. But the breathing thing was really important, I cannot say how much that helped. I could have given birth every weekend – pregnancy I hated, but I could do birth a million times. I felt really thrilled afterwards. I was on a total high for the first three days. I think it was a little bit about 'Aren't I amazing?' That I thought I'd done well. And I felt back to normal pretty soon afterwards, too. I didn't feel that I'd been through the wars.

11

Standing Birth

Lisa Joffe, 38, a teacher in Alexander Technique, gave birth to her second child Arthur standing up in a water pool in an NHS birth centre in Sussex, without the use of any drugs. Arthur was born two weeks overdue, with a lot of noise but only one push, weighing 9 lb 2oz.

I carried on teaching the Alexander Technique up until three months before Arthur was born, when the personal inter-action became too demanding. Alexander Technique is safe to take up and practise during pregnancy, which is actually a good time to work on your posture because the hormones soften the ligaments. The technique looks at the balance of your body and how it is organized. For example, looking at the relationship of the head, neck and back to the pelvis. Teachers use their hands to release gently unhelpful habits of tension and promote freedom in the joints and ease of movement. It also looks at how you can perform a simple movement with the least possible effort. So if I am reaching for my glass, I learn to do it while maintaining freedom in my neck, not clenching the glass, and using the least amount of energy. By doing that well, you minimize strain on your body.

I felt very grounded and stable during pregnancy, but it was a challenge, because the bump was pulling me forward and this could create strain in my lower back.

I had birthed my first child, Genna, 10 years previously in a pool with an independent midwife, and second time around I wanted to use my voice in a way that didn't cause me damage, because I was hoarse after Genna. I didn't know how to use that bellowing which I seem to do in labour without causing me pain and problems. With my second child, Arthur, I had a much clearer understanding about wanting to let myself make a lot of sound without forcing or causing strain. I wanted to make the sound in conjunction with what was happening, facilitating the birth rather than being separate. I felt much more connection with my whole body, a far greater sensitivity to myself this time around.

I was two weeks over my due date when I started having contractions in an Indian restaurant at 9.30 p.m., and they were intense from the beginning. My husband Malcolm said 'I think we need to go to Crowborough Birthing Centre' where he was very keen I had the baby. He really wanted the extra support of a birth centre, after the first experience at home. There was a part of me that wanted to have the baby at home, but I felt a little bit more vulnerable in our new Brighton home, and so had cancelled the pool two weeks before my due date. I liked the Crowborough, and had met all the midwives there, but I was a little concerned about the length of the drive.

It took us 45 minutes to drive there in full labour, and as we drove I noticed the full moon as I was howling through my contractions. We got there and I could hardly walk, really crouched over. We got into the birthing room, which was empty, and I went down on my knees making all this sound, quite scared. I could hear the midwife saying 'Have you considered any form of pain-relief?' and I just thought 'I'm here for the water' and Malcolm started filling up the pool, becoming the water-temperature man. I got into the water, which immediately helped, and I was on all fours.

The midwife who met us on arrival was the one person out of the group that I didn't feel very comfortable with. I felt she was anxious to get Arthur out, and that when he did come out he came out very suddenly, and there was no pacing of it. She was getting me to really push, and I just imagine that if I'd had someone who was more relaxed about the process of birthing, it might not have happened in such a dramatic way. But I was very raw at the time, and she really helped me through it. I felt a deep sense of support from her and Malcolm.

The contractions were coming every 10 minutes. My previous labour with Genna was really gradual, with an increasing intensity of contractions and shortening of the time between them, something I could understand. But this was much faster and more intense more quickly, although my waters never broke. I could feel this sensation where I didn't feel like I should push, but it was more like an enormous earthquake going on inside me. I was obviously in this transition stage for about half an hour, and my midwife said 'How do you feel about having your waters broken?' And I said 'That's fine,' because they had done the same with Genna.

I was there saying 'I don't think I can do it, I don't think I can do it' and the midwife was saying, 'You can do it, you are doing it' which made me think 'Yes, I am!' Then the midwife said 'Really push as if you are trying to do a poo,' which I hadn't done before with Genna. 'Really push into your anus,' she said, and I was really trying to do what she told me, but it didn't feel the best thing necessarily. I felt it was rather a crude instruction. I was a bit bewildered at that stage, but I knew I was minimizing strain on me and I was looking after myself.

The midwife then suggested that I get up off all fours and onto a low birthing stool that she put in the pool for me to sit on. So I sat on the stool for a while and then she said, 'Why don't you stand up?' And, as Malcolm helped me, in the motion of going from sitting to standing, with one contraction Arthur was born. I gave one push, and I couldn't believe it – there was this huge baby, he was real, like a sculpture, this person and it was so quick that the midwife at the edge of the pool just caught him from behind. She gave him to me, the umbilical cord was still attached and I sat down in the bath and held him. I was in a little bit of shock, and Arthur was crying, but there was a powerful moment of recognition between each other along with amazement that he was suddenly there. Gravity had been on our side and I suppose I had had him in the easiest way.

I remember holding him and thinking 'He looks very evolved, almost like a child rather than a baby.' Then he was wrapped up so he wouldn't get cold in the water, handed to Malcolm, and I went to lie down on the bed to deliver the placenta. I remember feeling in a heightened state of clarity, I felt tremendously alive, totally present and the feeling of experiencing the pain and that intensity was really important to me. I can't imagine what it would be like to give birth with an epidural. For me it was really important to feel everything, even though at times the contractions felt overwhelming and more than I could tolerate. For me, there is a rawness and intensity that brings with it an incredible feeling of exhilaration – almost like being born again.

On one level I was surrendering to the physical experience, and there was also an inevitability of motion. I felt Arthur was doing it his way. It was his journey out, and at that moment of birth he was separate, choosing his own form of expression.

12

Induction Birth

Lindsey Lloyd, 30, from Northampton, went into hospital soon after her waters had broken, and was asked to stay in to be induced after the baby's heart rate dipped a few times on the foetal monitor. Lindsey knew that an induction could lead to further intervention (with stronger contractions requiring more pain-relief) but weathered the experience well, enjoying her very first birth with the help of some relaxation and breathing techniques from her hypnobirthing classes.

My plan was to stay at home as long as possible, and not go into hospital until necessary. However, at 1 a.m. on Monday morning, the day before my due date, I woke up and my waters were leaking slightly. I wanted to go back to bed, but Tony started looking up what to do on the Internet, and wanted to ring the hospital an hour later. The hospital wanted me to come in to have a quick look before sending me back home, so we didn't take any bags and arrived around 3 a.m.

While monitoring the baby with a foetal monitor, the baby's heart rate dropped suddenly and the team put the flap down on the bed and started giving me oxygen for the baby's sake. The heart rate came back pretty quickly, but they wanted me to stay put for a while so they could monitor me further. They thought perhaps the baby was lying on his umbilical cord, causing his heart rate to dip. Because of this little situation, I was given a midwife to stay with me all the time while my husband Tony went home around 5 a.m., promising to be back at 9 a.m.

I wasn't really feeling any contractions around this time, so I put on my hypnobirthing music and Rainbow Relaxation tape to help me to get to sleep because I wasn't allowed off the bed. I started hypnobirthing classes after watching a programme about mind over matter on the television. The programme showed an experiment on camera where people screamed when given an electric shock after being told it was going to hurt; then, when given an electric shock after a placebo tablet and being told it *wasn't* going to hurt, they didn't flinch. I wondered whether using hypnosis might be possible for labour.

I found out about a local hypnobirthing instructor on the Internet and decided to try it out, paying £200 for four sessions. My husband Tony was supportive of my decision and, as the class was geared around including the partner and getting partners to relax alongside and hypnotize their labouring woman, he thought it was great [see page 90 for more details].

The baby's heart rate dipped a couple more times, so they put a monitor on the baby's scalp and announced that they wanted to get things moving and induce me because of the risk of infection. I also needed constant midwife attention.

As I said that I had wanted a natural birth and knew inductions could cause strong, fast contractions, they agreed to leave it until 11 a.m. to review their decision. By 11 a.m. I hadn't dilated any further than 2 cm, so they pushed me to go for the induction.

They hooked me up to a drip, and because I had made a fuss about being induced in the first place, they agreed to start off slowly with a low dose and then build it up. It did work and the contractions started, and by 1 p.m. I was in proper established labour. I had my hypnobirthing tapes, listened to the music and was doing my relaxation and affirmations while Tony stayed by the monitor telling me when the contraction had peaked and was going off. This was helpful because I'd adjust my breathing and I'd know when it was going to end.

I felt pretty in control, even though in the last couple of hours the contractions were really strong. I would feel them, but I wasn't scared or bothered by them. I had my eyes shut just lying there deeply relaxed, concentrated on my breathing and shutting out any distractions. Tony thought I was falling asleep! I would visualize slowly filling a balloon while breathing in, and visualize the balloon slowly drifting away when exhaling. I had to lie there anyway because I couldn't get off the bed with all the wires and monitors, I wasn't speaking to anyone, I was just getting on with it. When they checked me at 5 p.m. they said I was 8 cm dilated. And Tony thought I was asleep!

All of a sudden I felt that something was happening and I could feel the baby moving downwards. I sat upright and changed my breathing, breathing down – as opposed to slowly breathing in and out. The different breathing helps the descent of the baby. Then the midwife who had been with me through most of established labour examined me and said, 'You can start pushing now.' I decided to go with the midwife, rather than the breathing, and that felt right for then. The midwife didn't understand the breathing techniques, to her I was panting and not pushing, and I took a decision to go with whatever she said.

I had about four or five contractions to push with, and then there was one long contraction. She said, 'Do you want to have another push?' as the contraction subsided, and I did, and in one really quick moment the baby's head, shoulders and arms all came out. The midwife wasn't ready and had to shout for someone to come in. After a final little push, in a first labour lasting just under six hours, our healthy baby boy was born weighing 7 lb 3 oz. We named him Tom.

I had a little bit of a tear, and felt rather amazed that I had had this baby and hadn't had any pain-relief. I felt proud and pleased with myself rather than emotional. If anyone had asked me whether I'd do it again, at that moment I would have said 'Yes!' The funny thing was I had gas and air while having my stitches because it was painful, yet I had just given birth with no pain-relief.

I wasn't tired after the birth, and Tom was a very calm baby. Months later he is still a chilled-out baby who only cries when he's hungry, and I put that quality down to the birth. I also feel it was nice to prove everyone wrong. Everybody said when I told them about hypnobirthing that I would change my mind once I got into the hospital and be screaming for pain-relief, and it didn't happen like that. Everything you see on the telly about birth and everyone you speak to about birth always says, 'It's horrendous!' But all I did was learn a few techniques and had a really good labour. I even enjoyed it.

For more birth stories from mothers who used hypnobirthing techniques, visit the website www. hypnobirthing.co.uk.

13

Hoot Hoot Hout Birth

Lisa Collins had a 'back' labour and epidural for her first birth. For her second birth three years later, she was 30, living in Spain with her husband and son Joshua, and running a Children's Activity Camp. Here she describes being focused on the birth from the moment that she found out that she was pregnant, and how she successfully got through labour with breathing techniques and a determination to ignore Spanish hospital protocols.

My first son Joshua was born in hospital when I was 26, after a long 'back' labour, and I was grateful for the help of the midwives in the NHS who gave me an epidural to help things along. I didn't know any breathing techniques to help me dislocate from the pain, in fact I didn't know much about anything to do with the labour part of the pregnancy as I hadn't really focused on it until the last couple of weeks before his due date. I loved my pregnancy, and perhaps subconsciously avoided the whole pain aspect and, because I had trained as an actress, I convinced myself that I could wing labour on 'drama' breaths on the day.

So, when I became pregnant again, this time living in Spain, I began to focus on the labour from day one, seeing the 9 months as preparation for that 'crowning' moment. This was particularly important because I was thankfully bombarded with ex-pat mums eager to tell me all the things to expect from a Spanish hospital birth, such as: 'They'll make you lie down' or 'They'll want to put an IV drip into your arm, and that'll flow some sugary solution into your system which will speed up your contractions.' Or 'The IV drip means that the doctors can put you under general anaesthetic easily, should they need to ... which they often do.' I decided I wanted to be in as much control as possible and, having started yoga the previous year, I enlisted the help of my yoga teacher, Jenny, to prepare me.

I practised yoga daily throughout my pregnancy and attended Jenny's classes twice a week. Furthermore, when she began a Hatha Yoga meditation class I also went and 'blissed' out in that (nothing better than a good meditation class to connect with the baby growing inside you). I found all the poses to be beneficial, especially the inverted poses: Dog, Headstand and particularly Shoulderstand. [Don't try these at home without a qualified yoga teacher.] Any pose where my legs were raised higher than my heart seemed to create lots of space between the baby and myself. I was able to really connect with the idea that this was a separate human being growing inside me. Furthermore, in the last few weeks the Shoulderstand seemed to alleviate a lot of the pressure on my internal organs, which somehow enabled me to breathe more deeply and so relax.

At the end of the first trimester I began to drink raspberry-leaf tea – a yoga book had told me of its benefits – as it strengthens the uterus in pregnancy for labour and aids contractions. Although you are advised to increase the quantity in gentle increments, by the end of my pregnancy I was on at least six cups a day.

At the beginning of the third trimester I began one-hour breathing classes with Jenny, twice a week after yoga classes. She taught me three types of breath to use during labour:

1) A quiet thin breath ... breathing in through your nose, imagining your breath going down into your tummy like a piece of string and blowing out through your mouth gently and continuously. She said this breath was to be used as labour started, and through earlier milder contractions, to maintain focus, keep calm and reserve energy. It was also to be employed in the middle and end of the first stage of labour and into the second before bearing down, again to keep calm and relaxed, and again to reserve energy for the stronger contractions.

2) The second breath is a chest breath called 'Hoot Hoot Hout' breath. It is a strong breath into the chest, and as you breathe out equally strongly you literally say, 'Hoot Hoot Hout' – the 'Hout' being the positive affirmation that you are breathing the baby out. The idea is that by only breathing into your chest, you are dislocating yourself from the abdomen area, thus from the area where the baby is doing the work, and thus from the pain. This was

the most useful breath I learned. It was the breath that enabled me to birth my baby Jesse naturally

3) The third breath was a throat breath [sometimes called 'panting' like a dog]. It is where you only breathe fast and furiously as far as your throat and out again continuously, thus filling your head with a ton of oxygen. It was to be used in the last stages of the second stage of labour to dislocate even further from the pain and aid the pushing. To be honest I never really mastered that one, and although my memory is a bit hazy, I'm sure I carried on using a lot of Hoot Hoot Hout at that point.

In the last month of my work with Jenny she would make me practise 'mock' labours. She would make me imagine contractions had begun and then we would practise all the different breaths. In the early stages of this rehearsal she advised me to sit as still as possible, using Breath 1 quietly and calmly. As the 'mock' contractions heightened she encouraged me to walk around as much as possible in between contractions, and then when indicated I would go into Breath 2 (Hoot Hoot Hout). Jenny encouraged me to lean against walls, tables, chairs, anything to breathe it out more easily. *One of the best bits of information she gave me was that the worst contractions last only one and a half minutes.* This was really useful when I was actually in labour, as I remember thinking several times: 'This is agony but I've only a minute to go!' Jesse was born on his due date, and at about 5 p.m. the previous afternoon I went into labour whilst swimming, which had also been a big part of my pregnancy. I loved to lie on the warm sand on the beach face down, with a big hole scooped out for my huge stomach. Heaven. I knew this time, however, that something was happening because my body suddenly went light and I felt far away, like I was moving around on cotton wool. And although I felt calm and relaxed, I also knew that I wanted to get home.

My husband Liam and I were running a Children's Activity Camp, and he got back from work at about 6 p.m. to start timing contractions. They were already 5 minutes or so apart. I drank loads of raspberry-leaf tea and in between contractions was calm and still. By 10 p.m. I was walking about and leaning on furniture Hoot Hoot Houting away. We rang Jenny at around 1 a.m. and left for the hospital soon after. I remember sitting in the back of the car – Jenny and Liam chatting in the front – and suddenly realizing that my contractions had stopped. We were halfway to the hospital (20 minutes away) and no sign of a contraction anywhere. I panicked slightly and meekly suggested that it might be a false alarm. But my birthing partners decided we should go to the hospital anyway. (I later realized that I had been in transition from the first to the second stage of labour in the car, a time when contractions often stop for up to 20 minutes).

We arrived at the hospital and, as I got out of the car, my waters broke. Contractions started to kick in fast and furiously, and as I walked from the car to the hospital door I had at least two or three. As I slowly made my way up the hospital corridor, I stopped to have many a loud and dramatic Hoot Hoot Hout contraction along the way, leaning on every bit of wall I could find. Hospital orderlies were fussing around me trying to get me to sit in a wheelchair so that they could get me to the delivery room quickly, but Jenny staved them off, saying: '*Quieres Andar!*' ('She wants to walk!'). The walk must have taken a good half hour. When I got to the labour room I was immediately put on a bed, and then had to argue, in between contractions, with the doctor not to put an IV drip in my arm, and to insist that my husband could be present for the birth (that's another thing Spanish hospitals didn't encourage – husbands and birth partners were not allowed). At this point I was told I was 7 cm dilated and would be there for a while. More arguing ensued and about 20 minutes later I was checked again and found to be fully dilated. Arguing stopped, and my husband and the doctor walked me to the birthing room. Once again I was put on a bed. After several pushes lying on my back, and with an overwhelming desire to bear down, Jesse was born at 3 a.m. I was given an episiotomy, perhaps because ultimately there was no time to argue about what position to give birth in. However, I remember when Jesse was born he just opened his eyes, looked around, and shut them again. He made no sound until the doctor took a little blood from his ankle, when he gave a little cry, opened his eyes and then shut them again. He seemed calm and connected. He was then whipped off by nurses for routine checks and injections (I'd been warned about this, too, so wasn't surprised) and as I waited for him back in the ward I felt wide awake and elated. A few minutes later I once again ignored hospital protocol and went off in search of my beautiful little boy – *guapo blancito*, as the nurses called him.

14

IVF Birth

Jenny Cox, 34, set out to have her triplets by C-section and ended up birthing them normally in hospital. Jenny chose St George's Hospital in south London for her delivery because of its large Special Care Unit (triplet babies are usually born prematurely because of lack of space in the womb), and she had planned a Caesarean according to hospital policy. As it was, she went into labour spontaneously at 32 weeks and five days, giving birth to Sarah first (4 lb 10oz), Jake second (4 lb) and Martha third (3 lb 15 oz).

One of the things I wanted was for all the babies to be in the same hospital, and I chose St George's because it has one of the largest neonatal units in the country. You hear stories of triplet babies being split up into different hospitals at birth, and I didn't want that for mine.

When I went for my first consultancy appointment I was very pleased, they looked after me fantastically. St George's looks crummy and falling apart, but when it comes down to specialist medical care it is one of *the* places to go. I was told about the birth plan at the first appointment. They had been quite bossy about insisting on a Caesarean, but I wasn't too bothered. The whole IVF conception process had not been too natural, so I thought 'Why change anything now?' I was booked in for a Caesarean at 34 weeks, and it was highly recommended that I spend some time in the hospital during the pregnancy, because they say that periods of complete rest help to delay the birth. They told me I had two milestones to reach – 28 weeks and 32 weeks – and I got past them both.

My waters broke at 32 weeks and 5 days. I had my bag packed and called from the car with my husband Will to say 'It's happening'. My consultant was in Australia, and the consultant on call came and had a look and said, 'Yes you have gone into labour because your waters have broken, but you're not at all dilated.' I never thought I'd go into labour, because I'd never thought I'd have a natural birth. I'd been to the hospital antenatal classes but I hadn't really paid much attention, and certainly not listened about how you push babies out.

They said 'Right. What we'll do, because nothing is going to happen for a little while, is give you another steroid injection (I'd already had a course), we'll book the time for your Caesarean today and we'll contact the neonatal unit to see when they'd like to have you all.' So they were very calm about the whole thing, and even suggested Will went home.

The time was about 2.30 a.m. in the morning, and Will was told to come back in around 7 a.m. At 7 I had the show [a plug of mucus] and the contractions started. Will was back by then so he didn't miss anything, the midwives came and had a look and said, 'We know you're having contractions, you're still not very dilated, the neonatal unit has said they would like you this afternoon.' My Caesarean was booked for 2 p.m., and I met the consultant and his team and the anaesthetist.

I had a midwife in my room with me the whole time, she hardly ever popped out, and was only looking after me. I'd met her before, she was around the same age as me, and I liked her, she was funny. The contractions started coming and they were painful – I didn't expect them to be so painful so soon. She spoke to the anaesthetist about whether I could have any pain-relief, and he suggested only gas and air. She didn't think I should have gas and air because I'd be huffing and puffing on that from 9 a.m. in the morning until 2 p.m. in the afternoon and thought I might feel awful on it.

So I was in agony, not listening to anything anybody said. At that point I had two midwives, one for me and one for the babies. One went out for a few minutes, and then came back and said, 'You look like you're trying to push,' and I said, 'I don't know what I'm doing.' So she sort of described it and I said, 'Yes … yes I am.' She left suddenly, and I later learned that she ran down the corridor crying out, 'Triplet mum is trying to push!' The doctor appeared suddenly and said 'Oh! You're 10 cm dilated, we better give you a Caesarean now!' This had all happened in the space of one hour – which explains why the contractions had been so painful.

We knew at this stage that baby Sarah was head-down and ready to go, Jake in the middle, moving around the whole time, and Martha was transverse [lying across]. I knew the sexes of the babies – I thought we'd have enough surprises with triplets. The midwife rushed me out of my nightie and within 2 minutes I was being wheeled into the operating theatre on my back, with two monitors on and four pads – one for the contractions and one for each baby. When I got into the operating theatre, everyone was already there – lined up and ready. And this is why I think St George's is so fantastic, because everyone was ready to go in less time it took the midwife to run outside and say, 'Triplet mum is trying to push!'

The needle for my spinal block went into my back, which did cause a few problems later on because I couldn't feel to push. Then the consultant I'd seen before had a look and said 'Oh! Your daughter's almost out! We can't do the Caesarean.' If the head has only just started to come down, they can push it back up again, but her head was so far down that they couldn't.

I couldn't feel a thing, and he announced, 'You're going to have to push her out.' I was scared. I didn't know how to do a normal birth and the midwives had to explain what 'pushing' was to me. I was worried for my safety and the babies, because this was the reason they gave me for planning a Caesarean birth. I remember lying on the table thinking 'Oh my God, what if all four of us are going to die?' But everyone was being very calm.

I couldn't feel what I was doing, and in fact Sarah needed forceps to help her out. Sarah was the biggest and the eldest and most determined to come out. I think she thought she'd had enough in there. The consultant then said that Jake was presented the right way round, which they knew from the scans that they were doing on me as the birth happened. So the consultant said, 'You might as well push him out while you are at it.' So out came Jake with the help of a ventouse. I had to wait until the contractions started again, and there was half an hour between Sarah and Jake being born.

I wasn't really very aware of what was going on, I was finding it all quite hard work and all very mechanical, and I couldn't really see much. I had drips in my arms, and my legs in the stirrups. Jake and Sarah were both fine, they were shown to me before being taken off to their incubators, but Martha was not yet ready to come out, her waters had yet to break and they were concerned about her heart rate – she'd been in too long with all the contractions going on. She was also in an odd position, she was transverse. There was talk of a C-section but I said, 'Oh no, we've got this far, can't she come out naturally as well?' So the consultant said he'd attempt to turn her around manually into the breech position, to birth her that way. The midwife told me afterwards that if I hadn't had my spinal block that 'internal version' would have been very painful.

Martha wasn't so well when she was born, she wasn't shown to me and was whisked away to be resuscitated, with all the paediatricians diving over her incubator. Then I heard her yell, and the obstetrician said 'There you are, that's a relief isn't it?'

I felt awful after the birth, very tired, particularly for the first few hours. I didn't have an episiotomy, but I had had a tear and was in a lot of pain when the spinal block wore off. Apparently I had lost a lot of blood and they wanted to give me a blood transfusion, but I'd had enough and refused it. They said I would have felt a lot a better if I'd had one. With the contractions starting at 8 a.m. I was all tidied up and finished with by 1 p.m. I must say that the midwives were practically cheering the consultant by the end of it.

So many nice things about the birth on reflection. I came home two weeks before the babies did,* and I could drive. If I woke up at 4 a.m. and wanted to see them, I could get in a car and go (new mothers are advised not to drive for six weeks after Caesarean births). Sometimes I would drop in just for a few minutes.

I stayed for a week in the hospital. It was nicer to be in because I was nearer to the babies and I was trying to get all the expressing sorted out. I breastfed for eight weeks with the help of a breastfeeding counsellor, and Jake was fed exclusively on my milk because anything else made him sick. The girls had what was left over because I didn't produce enough for all three.

* Because the babies were born at 33 weeks, their sucking reflex, which kicks in between 34 and 36 weeks,

had yet to develop, so they needed to be tube-fed. The babies also needed to learn to maintain their body temperature before they were allowed home at 36 weeks.

15

Breech Birth

Rachael Wheatley, 38, was 14 weeks pregnant when she hired her independent midwives in Bristol for her second baby. At her 20-week scan she discovered that the placenta was quite low, so she was rescanned at around 34 weeks – only to find that the placenta had moved up, but that the baby was lying in extended breech (legs stretched out either side of the body). Her baby boy, Cormac, was born normally in February 2004, weighing 7 lb 11 oz.

I hired my independent midwives for the second birth after I saw an advert in the local NCT magazine. I had had my first child in hospital and I had felt her birth was very 'managed'. She was posterior, my labour was augmented, I was given an epidural and the baby was born with the help of a ventouse. I felt very distant from it all, and I didn't want to go into hospital and have the same experience again, and so was hoping for a home birth second time around. I wanted to know exactly who was going to be there to help me birth my baby and to have built up trust with a known midwife during my pregnancy.

When I found out the baby was breech, I tried everything: acupuncture, moxibustion (see page 48), homoeopathic remedies, swimming and doing handstands in the pool. I even tried a chiropractor and kneeling with my bum in the air, but the baby remained resolutely breech. One of the midwives was a great believer in fate, and that things would work out, and as it turned out I was so glad I hired independent midwives, because I wouldn't have had the choices I had if they weren't.

I was very upset about the baby being breech; I felt that all my plans had gone awry. We read a lot of articles and the new book by Benna Waites [*Breech Birth*, Free Association Books 2003] and looked at the Term Breech Trial, gold-standard research done comparing the outcomes for mother and baby for Caesarean and vaginal breech delivery. This trial showed that it was several times safer to have a Caesarean than a medically-managed birth (which often involves the use of epidural, forceps, being on your back with stirrups). Other evidence suggested that a natural breech birth was possible, but the best outcomes were with experienced practitioners and a 'hands-off' approach – where you don't touch or manoeuvre the baby unless absolutely necessary, and then only very gently.

We spent two or three weeks going through the decision-making process. Should we have a Caesarean, a medically-managed breech, an active breech birth at home (if the hospitals weren't supportive), or find a hospital that would support a normal breech birth? My instinct was to go for an active breech birth because I didn't want to be denied the experience of birth, or to have to look after a new baby and toddler after a Caesarean – but, I agonized, was I being selfish?

A lot of doctors overplay the risks of breech birth and underplay those of Caesareans. We felt there are risks in a normal head-down birth that aren't necessarily mentioned, whereas with a breech birth everyone emphasizes the risks. While it is true that there are some possible complications with breeches, if properly managed we're still talking small. We saw two consultants, one in Bristol and one in Bath, to talk about external cephalic version (ECV) [a procedure where an experienced practitioner turns the baby manually by manipulating the mother's stomach] and about how they would manage a breech birth.

In Bristol I came away very upset; the consultant talked about the risk of the placenta coming away or the cord coming around the baby's neck in ECV, and he even talked about how the possibility of decompression and recompression of the head during birth could lead to the baby's head 'exploding'. If we didn't know better, we would have been scared into a C-section.

The consultant in The Royal United Hospital in Bath, Dr Rick Porter, was much more supportive. He was positive about ECV as a safe procedure and agreed that, although there were some small risks, he would be happy to go for an active breech birth. My midwives could also practise in the Bath hospital. So we came away thinking that if we were going to have it, we would have it in Bath. My husband Rob was keen on going to hospital for a breech, he was also thinking about a Caesarean until I gave him Benna Waites' book to read and he felt more reassured.

By 38 weeks we settled on an active breech birth in Bath with no doctors, no paediatricians in the room to whisk the baby away (although they would be outside if needed) and just my midwives and the independent midwife Mary Cronk, who was experienced in breech birth. If labour didn't progress well we agreed we'd go for a C-section. I felt relieved, calm and confident, assured that this was the right decision for us and our baby, and that we were in the best possible hands with our birth attendants.

I went overdue, but Mary Cronk didn't seem to be worried. At five days' overdue I finally went into labour with a few twinges, like mild period pains, coming every 10 or 15 minutes from 4 a.m. until 9 in the morning. Then things went up a gear and it became more intense, and we left after noon for the hospital. The journey was easy enough, with me contracting every 10 minutes over the half hour it took to arrive. Then I had two strong contractions as I walked into hospital. We'd brought quite a lot of stuff in, we wanted to be surrounded by things that were ours, we had a birthing ball, photos of our daughter, pillows, cushions, food, a tape recorder with music and my hospital bag.

As I was getting settled into the room, Mary Cronk arrived and after a while the midwives withdrew to let us get on with it. At about 2 p.m., an hour after we arrived in hospital, it got very intense. I was pacing up and down the room, closing my eyes and visualizing my cervix and saying, 'Open.' My husband was there, I'd lean against him and have the contraction, or use the bed or ball to lean on. I had a TENS machine, which had been helpful early on but I kept forgetting to turn it up. Labour was building over a few hours, and I must have reached transition at the stage when I felt 'I can't cope.'

Soon after I had two or three milder contractions and went very quiet. Then my waters broke and quite soon after I wanted to push. I had missed that feeling with my first baby because of the epidural; it was a very powerful feeling – and a relief to push through the contractions and do something with the pain.

I was beside the bed on my hands and knees [Mary Cronk calls this 'the Christian prayer position'] for most of the second stage, but early on they wanted to see a little more progress, so I squatted to give it more 'welly'. But I found squatting quite hard, and it would have been too much of a stretch for the perineum, so I got back into the Christian prayer position, with talk of a 'conversion to Islam' [nose on the floor and bum in the air] later if necessary. The baby's bottom eventually 'rumped' [breech-speak for 'crowned'] and good progress was then made in the next 7 minutes.

The general view is that a breech baby should be born within 15 minutes of 'rumping'. I could feel myself being stretched for the time that the whole length of the body came down [sometimes called 'laying the golden egg' because the shape of the baby is a perfect oval until a leg drops down]. One leg came out, then the other dropped down. Then the arms dropped down soon after, then the chin, mouth and half the nose. The midwife then performed something called the Smellyvite manoeuvre where the midwife gently touches the baby's cheekbones and flexes the neck forward and the head comes out. Cormac's breathing was a bit snuffly at first and he seemed a bit drowsy, so he took a little time to come round, but pinked up nicely.

I felt amazed, dazed, relieved. Rob clamped the cord once it had stopped pulsating and I delivered the placenta 20 minutes afterwards in a reclining position.

I felt very smug and very proud the day after. I'd done something that not many women do – and I felt elated. I had no baby blues afterwards, as I had with my first daughter. If you have a positive birth experience it really helps set you up for looking after a small baby. I had wanted to be a part of the birth, not distant, and it felt empowering. I had wanted to do it, but I had a hangover from my first birth of 'Can I do it?' I was proud that my body worked and did what it was supposed to do.

People have to make the decisions that are right for them, but shouldn't be scared to seek a second opinion. I went against mainstream medical opinion, but was backed by experienced practitioners in a supportive environment. Having an independent midwife made a difference to our decision about having an active breech birth. Even aside from this decision, the independent midwifery model is first class, and every woman should have the right to that type of care.

16

Twin Birth

Gaia Pollini was 32 when she gave birth to her twins at home in southwest London. As someone who teaches rebirthing, a teaching centred around breathing, she felt that it was important to bring her two babies into the world in the most spiritual way possible. They were her first babies, and after all the careful planning she had an ecstatic birth that prompted her to set up ante-natal classes soon after called Birthing with God.

I was six weeks pregnant when I went for an independent midwife. I had some bleeding the first week I found out I was pregnant, which is how I found out that I was carrying twins because of the scan at St George's. It was fantastic, because when you bleed the first thing you think of is a miscarriage, and then we walked out knowing it was twins. I personally think it is better to know everything so you can go through the process of letting go. I have read of people who were part of a vanishing twin and that have felt all their life that there was something missing, and then did past-life regression work and realized that were part of a team that never was.

After the scan I went to my NHS doctor to find out what twins meant, and she said, 'You'll have to get scans every two weeks, and have a hospital birth: we'll monitor you here and monitor you there.' It's not that we had been thinking about birth – I was adamant about natural birth because of my work as a Rebirther, and it was really important to me, so I got put off straight away. She was quite harsh. In a way, I thank her because she got me to run away very quickly from the hospital option.

We couldn't get a home birth on the NHS, so we got an independent midwife when eight weeks pregnant. I interviewed three sets of independent midwives. The first two sets of midwives I interviewed were pushing for a hospital birth because of insurance, but they did say there would be a birthing room and we wouldn't be disturbed. They nearly persuaded me on it because I thought if independent midwives were saying that then insurance must be necessary. However, when the final set of independent midwives said they had no insurance, and why not opt for a home birth, I was drawn to them. 'Let's see how the pregnancy goes,' they said, 'If you go to term and there are no problems let's go for a home birth, if you don't, and there are, we won't.' That was great. It was really interesting because when the NHS doctor said, 'Hospital birth' I thought, 'She's just saying that,' but when the independent midwives said, 'Hospital birth', I trusted them for it. My independent midwives were quite excited about doing a home birth with twins as well.

I was so glad not to have to have anything to do with hospitals for the rest of my pregnancy. We knew from the early scan that the babies had two placentas and two sacs. Then two weeks before the second scan was due I had quite strong bleeding for two days, so I got scared, but we had a scan and saw everything was OK. But I asked for no nuchal scan and the guy nearly bit my head off. He was actually horrible, really aggressive, saying 'Why don't you want a nuchal scan? Why are you here then?' He just couldn't believe it and was quite scary really. It was like an interrogation. We had to really explain ourselves. We were worried about the bleeding and it wasn't any way to treat a person lying on a bed vulnerable and prone. So that was the last scan I had.

I loved my pregnancy, it was fantastic, it was a real journey. I was very open and I wasn't always feeling great – I had lots of stuff from the past that came up about my mum, relationships, my relationship with my parents, how I was treated as a child, and that was a lot of up and down, but it was very healing. It was really beautiful and I really let myself be. If I felt down I cried and if I felt great I laughed, it felt quite full-on – all the things that came up got resolved really quickly, the love of being pregnant can cause you to be stronger to be with yourself. In my course, when I was seven-and-a-half months' pregnant, I did a sweat lodge (although they tell you not to go near the heat) because the heat is really healing and purifying in my work. I really experimented.

I actually had a sense that my growing children were loving it. They were loving experiencing the world early. I think these babies are living beings the moment they are conceived, and what your experience of the world is, they experience. And I think they love you experiencing the world because they are experiencing it, too. And every time I was doing something out of the ordinary, like experiencing the heat and the cold, I would connect with them and ask if it was OK, and I always got this big 'Yes' back.

I would say the most important thing, particularly the most important thing for me, was to stay away from other people's fears. I did not want to be near anybody going 'Oh, my God this' or 'Oh my God that', and that's why I didn't go to the hospital or near some of my friends. We just said, 'We know what we're doing, we don't need your opinion.'

I hardly had any negative feelings myself, I knew that I didn't want the babies to come early [due to the extra weight and size of twins, the womb decides there is no more room at the end of pregnancy, and twins arrive early more often than not]. I wanted them to come on time, in fact they were five days' late. I'd always visualize that I would give birth at term, so every time anybody said, 'When's your due date?' and I would tell them and they'd reply, 'Oh, they are going to be early because they are twins,' I'd say 'No, mine are not!' I visualized a lot, I'd talk to the twins a lot, I used any positive tools. I filled myself with the excitement. I expected to have a fantastic pregnancy, I expected to have a fantastic birth, and that's what I got. I had to force myself, towards the end of pregnancy, to imagine having to go into hospital so that it wouldn't be too much of a shock if it happened, because up until then it had never even crossed my mind.

The midwives really helped, they kept this energy up, they created a shield around me. All the nervousness from the rest of the world, they take it on. I think I would have found it a lot harder without that support.

So I got to 40 weeks and 4 days. I hardly had any Braxton Hicks [early contractions]. I was quite heavy, and I was not ready until the day I went into labour. I didn't get into the nesting thing until the last two weeks, I didn't get any of my home birth things. Annie Francis [one of Gaia's midwives] kept telling me off because three weeks before the birth I still didn't have my plastic sheets! I still had to do some letting go, I had the pool upstairs and I did a lot of relaxation and breathing. I hired the pool two weeks before the birth and I used it for the last week. I would do some breathing, which was wonderful because you are weightless.

A couple of days before the birth I was doing my wedding album. I put it away, thinking I had nothing else to do, and thought 'Now I am ready.' The next day I went into labour. My waters leaked a little, and after two or three hours I started to feel a few contractions. It was early in the morning, about 5 a.m., but I could feel them pretty well from the beginning, they were quite mild, and I timed them and they were about 6 or 7 minutes' apart. When John got up I called the midwife, and she was pleased because she said that if I hadn't gone into labour by then, they were going to send me for a scan.

At that stage the babies were really low. They were really ready to come out. So I called my other midwife, Alice, and she said she'd come lunchtime, but I wanted her to come then! (I felt I wanted someone knowledgeable around, because the contractions were quite strong.) I had also planned for my friend Monica to come, another Rebirther who was going to support me and be a supporter for John. She was a close friend and had done the breath work, and was absolutely fantastic.

By the time the midwife came around midday, I thought the contractions were quite strong. I think that the worst thing that happened to me was that two of my close friends had had babies a few months earlier, and one had an 8-hour labour and the other a 10-hour labour, so I was convinced I'd be the same. I thought by midday I was halfway there. The midwife said, 'You seem to be doing very well,' but there was hardly any dilation.

I had a 24-hour labour in the end. I think I was well prepared, but the contractions were much stronger than I'd imagined. I never thought about pain-relief, I was so prepared for every-thing to work out and to not take any drugs, and three days after the birth someone asked me 'Did you take gas and air?' and I hadn't even thought about it. I think that was the effect of arriving at the birth so positive and thinking 'It's going to be fine whatever happens.' So it was more about keeping myself on the positive track – however intense the contrac-tions were.

I was very present, and that's what the breathing does, because I was breathing very fully and when tension and fear comes in you just let go of it. So I never went through a 'What am I going to do now? It's 20 hours!' There were only a couple of times that I felt like crying and was like, 'I can't do it!' And it wasn't so much that I couldn't do it, I had just had enough. And as soon as that feeling came on, I was so aware that I couldn't afford to be there, and I think that is when people take drugs. I can imagine why people end up going in for Caesareans at that point, there was about 20 seconds when I let myself go in for the negative turn-off, and if you go down there then it's much harder to run back to the positive. It's much easier to stay in the positive – like anything in life, when you go into a ditch, it takes the extra effort to get out again.

I didn't want anything to drink, the midwife gave me Rescue Remedy, they brought all the glucose drinks but I didn't want them. It was really full-on, I was going into every room in the house, the only room I didn't go into was the living room at the front of the house. I think I quite liked to be at the back of the house, and laboured a lot in the bathroom. I had some showers around 15 hours into labour. And the midwife tried to move me around a bit more, because you can get a bit settled, and you can find comfort during the discomfort. So she asked me to move and we did going up and down the stairs. And I did a lot of 'in' breath and 'out' breath, with relaxation on the 'out' breath. We said 'Yes' a lot on the 'out' breath, I had my husband and friend saying 'Yes' a thousand times, to counterbalance any 'Oh my God.' When you say 'Yes' your body opens up, and so it was 'Yes, yes, yes!' like sex. I don't know what the neighbours thought!

And even during the strongest contractions I was also saying 'More, more, more' and that really helped me, it made me feel like a heroine to ask for more. So we were using all that stuff.

With the birthing pool, when it came to it, I didn't fancy it at all. I really wanted to have my feet on the ground. I had heard some stuff about hot water slowing down contractions, and something may have been going on in my head about keeping on track. It had already taken so long, and I couldn't bear it to go on longer than it should. I really felt capable. I think I had about 10 hours of contractions with no gap. I could feel them slow down and then a new one start. Slowly I was dilating all the time, I never really got stuck, it was just slow. The first child was head-down, but was turning around.

So it was hard, they never did any monitoring because I didn't want it, and then I didn't want to know how many centimetres dilated I was either. When the midwife Annie arrived about 3 a.m., labour was getting really active, I had been on my feet and I was 7 cm then. She suggested that I go to the pool to try and relax and be still, and almost sleep. And it did slow down but they were not as close together and she showed me how to use the 'out' breath more. She also explained what was happening inside; that helped a lot. She explained that if I relaxed in the lower muscles then the baby might have a chance to move how he needed to. So that really kept me going, because by then it had been really high energy. So I did a couple of hours in the pool, with both Monica and Annie with me.

Then I had this incredible urge to push, and they thought I wasn't ready. They got Alice up, John was asleep, and I was fully dilated and I think I knew because there was no stopping this urge to start pushing. And I loved the pushing. I'd do that any time. I think it was a fantastic release of energy from all that building up. However beautiful and holy you can make it, it is hard work. I used all the things that I had, and after 15 hours of it you just want to give birth. I had prepared for a beautiful birth and they asked me to get out of the pool, as we had agreed that beforehand, but I didn't want to. But I was in a difficult position, so I had to come out.

I loved the feeling of the baby coming down, and then it became really godly. I was talking to the baby, saying 'I really love you,' and I had no pain whatsoever in the final bit. The baby came really quickly, from the moment I started pushing I think it was 15 minutes. I was on my hands and knees, they caught him, and I had no cutting [episiotomy] or anything. It was Leone first. They caught him and gave him to John. And then I saw him. I looked at him and straightaway felt like pushing again. The incredible thing was that when they examined me 10 minutes after Leone was born, he [twin two] was head down – he just dived. And this was quite funny because we knew he was breech from about a month and a half after the birth.

Every time I got in touch with Arco [twin two] during the pregnancy, he always said 'Don't worry, I know what I'm doing, I'll be OK.' And the minute his brother came out, Arco dived down and was ready. And that was great. It was 11 minutes and it was quite easy. They clamped Leone's cord because of the second twin, and they cut the cord of Leone quite quickly and they left Arco's cord on because he wasn't breathing quite so hard. They had prepared me that the second twin can find the breathing a bit harder, and they had one of those little hand machines [to monitor and measure breathing]. I knew he wasn't breathing, but I just did not worry at all, there were three midwives there and I knew he was going to be all right. There was no panic there, not like in a hospital when there's something wrong. I could imagine all the manic things that could happen in hospital when people are running around and the mother then panics and the baby panics and it is a shock. But they were doing this thing, and I could sense there was no fear around.

Then he was breathing and I had them both, and I felt absolutely exhausted. The feeling of emptiness was so strong after all that breathing, I breathed strongly for 24 hours, and I felt quite breathless and like my organs were in a different place. And all my plans to light candles and get back into the pool, it was all I could do to hold the babies and try to breastfeed them.

So I was very tired, and I wanted to lie down, and they gave a bath to Arco (just under 6 lb) and Leone (7 lb 4 oz) – so they were good size. Arco was smaller with a wrinklier head, in the water he had the white stuff and vernix – shedding like a whole layer of skin. This was because he was a little over-due. They both started breastfeeding straight away and there was no tearing. It really couldn't have gone any better.

Gaia and John have now moved back to Italy and run a yoga retreat called The Hill That Breathes (www.the-hillthatbreathes.com). Gaia is still breastfeeding her three-year-old twins.

17

Epidural Birth

Allegra Huston was born and lived in Britain before moving to the US. She was 38 when she gave birth to her first child, Rafael Guevara, in Taos, New Mexico. Taos has the highest out-of-hospital birth rate in the States, and Allegra had put a lot of thought into planning for the birth she wanted. In the end, her baby was occupying a posterior position (the baby's back is against the mother's spine) which made her labour that much more prolonged and painful, with backache and more irregular contractions. After trying everything from visualization to having tennis balls jammed into her back, and with her blood pressure climbing, she had an epidural. The result was miraculous: she fell asleep and woke up 40 minutes later, ready to push the baby out.

I hadn't had my period for about six weeks, but I hate doctors so I didn't want to go to one, and I felt perfectly normal and that nothing was wrong with me. But when my period still didn't come I thought, well, something's wrong, I better go and see the doctor. She listened to my belly and said,

'You're pregnant!' I felt like such an idiot, like one of those high school girls who insists she never knew she was pregnant and gives birth in the ladies' loo on prom night.

At that point the doctor sent me off for a scan at the hospital. The first scan was all fine, so I arranged to be taken care of by an independent midwife, Julie Schochet, whom I'd known for a few years. I remember thinking once, watching her hula-hoop at a party, 'I should get pregnant just so Julie could be my midwife.' Because my blood pressure is a bit high normally, she had to get approval from the doctors at the Birth Centre to look after me, and they agreed that she would consult with them regularly. It started off being about 125 over 85 or 90. There is a law in the States that says that if your blood pressure is higher than 140 over 90, you cannot have an out-of-hospital birth. But I'm kind of phobic about hospitals, and I really didn't want to go there.

The great thing about being looked after by an independent midwife is the individual attention. Julie would come to my house every two weeks and spend maybe two hours. She was very big on vitamins and essential fatty acids and exercise. I walked and did yoga, which I would have been doing anyway, and I also joined a prenatal class. I don't like swimming in chlorinated pools, so I swam in the river, but by 7 months it was becoming too difficult. She also made me keep a record of everything I ate, because a diet high in protein can help keep blood pressure under control. But no matter what I did, my blood pressure kept creeping up. I had hypnotherapy, two massages a week, Chinese herbs, yoga, meditation, swimming, and still my blood pressure would not come down. Eventually they put me on drugs, but that didn't work either. Nothing made any difference. It was stuck on 150 over 110.

I didn't have any of the other symptoms of pre-eclampsia [a dangerous condition in pregnant women that is curable by immediate delivery of the baby], such as protein in the urine. I was convinced there was nothing really wrong with me, and still hoped for an out-of-hospital birth, but it was impossible. One of the main risks of high blood pressure is 'placenta abrupta' – where the pressure of the blood actually forces the placenta off the uterine wall – and it can be fatal for the baby.

As my due date approached Julie helped me decide on 'the team' who would be with me: Julie, my partner Cisco Guevara, and my friend Tara. Tara and Julie are also good friends. I had had an amnio, because of my age, and at 36 weeks the doctor sent me to the hospital for a scan, to check whether the baby was growing well, and for a foetal non-stress test, which measures the baby's heartbeat, to make sure he wasn't in any distress because of my blood pressure. The foetal non-stress test was repeated every week for the last month of my pregnancy.

The first time I was really nervous but, knowing how I felt, Julie came with me. Because all the birthing rooms were occupied, I had to have the non-stress test in the intensive care baby room, which was much more medical and completely freaked me out. Julie just climbed up and parked herself on the counter beside me, with her feet on the bed where I was lying. That was great, because she was so casual about it; there wasn't any of that tiptoeing around that makes hospitals so scary.

The last couple of times the hospital nurses put me in the room that would be mine when I came to have the baby. That helped me, because it was designed to be as be comfortable and relaxed-looking as possible. There is a little outdoor area and windows that you can open. You can go outside and walk up and down. They also allow you to decorate the room, bring in your own bedding, food and stereo. By the time I went into labour I was starting to feel very comfortable in the hospital – hypnotherapy also helped me in getting over my phobia – and Tara and I had a great time planning our interior décor. We decided to hang saris on the walls to cover the medical equipment, and started referring to the room as the Casbah.

What I came to value most about Julie was that she was open to both conventional and unconventional ways of doing things. If there was something that I asked her and she didn't know, she'd go and do the research. She would encourage me to ask her anything that I was afraid of, and to do affirmations such as 'I am strong, my body will open up like a flower' and 'The baby will be born smoothly and gently.' I am not a great person for doing that kind of thing, but it didn't feel foreign at all, it made a lot of sense (although I didn't write them up and put them on my fridge or bathroom mirror, which many people do). Julie also encouraged Cisco and me to do perineal massage. We used olive oil and it was surprisingly painful to do it properly, but it also felt so ridiculous that we would end up laughing. I would lie on the sofa and Cisco would watch TV over my shoulder. That was towards the end, during the last month. Though in the end I did tear a little, but I'm sure it was to do with the massage that I healed really easily and painlessly.

Julie came to all my doctor appointments with me. It was comforting to have her, both because we had grown close and because she shared my opinion that birth should not be medicalized if at all possible. When the doctor said 'I think we should do this' or 'I think we should do that,' I would turn to Julie and say, 'What do you think?' No matter how well the doctor is explaining it, you don't know because you've never been through it before. I knew that Julie had lots of experience, she knew exactly what I wanted and why I wanted it. Sometimes it would be a slightly awkward situation because doctors don't like to be second-guessed, so I would wait until the appointment was over and ask her what she thought once we were outside.

A few days before my due date, the doctor suggested inducing me slowly, because it looked as if I would go at least a week over term and my blood pressure was getting worrisome. Of course, I turned to Julie for her opinion. She said, 'Yes, I understand why she wants to induce you, and if she's going to do it slowly that's great, and if it takes four or five days that's fine, but don't let them put you on this stuff that really kicks in fast. That you don't want.' The doctors weren't using pitocin [syntocinon is the equivalent in the UK] at that point so that was fine, but it was nice to feel like Julie was a step ahead on what I wanted. I felt I could absolutely trust her judgement.

To induce, they used prostaglandin gel to make the cervix dilate. Midwives aren't accredited to do that, so the Birth Centre doctors had to do it in the hospital. You lie there for an hour, then you go home. They did this once on Thursday, not at all on Friday, and three times on Saturday, when I had one at 8 in the morning, one in the afternoon and one around 6 p.m. in the evening. They did it twice more on Sunday, and Julie gave me castor oil [a midwife's favourite to induce a baby] and I also went to the acupuncturist. Finally, I went into labour around 11 p.m. on Sunday night.

The prostaglandin gel makes you feel very crampy, like you are having a really bad period, and at first I thought the pain in my abdomen was just the result of the gel. Then I realized it was labour pains. I spent the night in the bath and called Julie at around 4 in the morning. Cisco was asleep and I didn't wake him up till after I had called Julie. I was handling it fine, but then the contractions turned into back labour. Julie suggested getting out of the bath and lying on the floor.

I was quite excited that I wasn't going to be pregnant anymore. I was tired of being pregnant, very sick of it by then, hot and uncomfortable. I wasn't scared about the birth, it was just something I had to do. I was hoping I was going to get through it without an epidural. I had read about epidural babies coming out drugged up and dozy, and also I wanted to have the full experience of birth, even though I knew it would be painful. Julie was accredited as a teacher of a method called Hypnobirthing, so she gave me and Cisco hypnobirthing classes (see page 90). It's all about concentrating on your breathing and not fighting the pain, relaxing so that your body can open smoothly.

Julie came to my house around 5 in the morning. She tried many techniques to relieve the back labour, including injecting sterile water underneath the skin into my lower back. Only the midwives know how to do this, not the doctors – later, in the hospital, I asked the doctor to do it (Julie was not allowed to treat me in the hospital, though she was allowed to be present) and she didn't know how. The injections cut the pain of the back labour completely for three hours, but it is like being stung by four hornets at once (it's the second-most painful thing I've ever experienced, back labour being the first!). It took the pain away to such a degree that I even went to sleep, and when I woke up we went to the hospital, around 10 a.m., with contractions about 5 minutes apart.

By the time I got to the hospital my contractions had gone back to around 7 minutes apart, but my waters broke as I got out of the car, so that put a clock on everything. I was only 2 cm dilated. For about two hours the contractions were 5 minutes apart. I was perfectly comfortable, sitting on the floor doing yoga to cope with the pain. Cisco and Tara were with me. We had decided what food we wanted to eat, because Julie is very big on making sure you have food to eat in labour, to keep up your strength. We had fruit, salad, tabouleh – they even had a fridge in the hospital room. I felt incredibly lucky to be at a hospital that had been 'trained' by the midwives, so the nurses who worked there were focused on the comfort and concerns of the mother.

The doctor was a little worried about the baby, and there were couple of moments when she was definitely preparing me for a C-section, but we stuck with it. They were monitoring his heart rate with pads [foetal monitors] and it seemed to drop quite dramatically, but they said that maybe the pads were picking up my heart rate, not his, so they put an internal monitor on his scalp. It turned out that the pad had indeed been picking up my heart rate, so I was saved.

As my contractions showed no sign of speeding up, and the clock was ticking because my waters had broken, the doctors decided to put me on pitocin (syntocinon here in the UK – used to augment contractions]. I was nervous about this, but Julie supported the doctors and convinced me it was the right thing to do. The pitocin made the pain in my back much worse, and one contraction seemed to run right into the next, with no break between them to get my strength back. I phoned my yoga teacher and she said, 'Tennis balls – get someone to push some tennis balls into your lower back', so Tara went off and got some. They had to take turns because it was so hard on the hands of whoever was jamming the tennis balls into my back!

By the middle of the afternoon, 18 hours since labour started, I was only 3 cm dilated – an increase of only 1 cm. My
blood pressure had gone up to 160 over 120, so the doctor
insisted that something had to be done to lower it, because
of the risk to both the baby and me. The choices were a Caesarean, an epidural, or some other blood pressure-lowering
drug. I was very sure that I didn't want a Caesarean and, even
though I hadn't wanted an epidural, I was in such agony that
it seemed like the right thing. I thought that perhaps the
stress of the pain was preventing my cervix from dilating.

Before the epidural I had this focus on whoever was in front
of me. When Julie did the sterile water injections, Tara held
both my hands and I got through the pain by totally focusing
on her. Cisco was doing all the stuff that we had learned at
hypnobirthing, saying 'You can do it! You can do it! You are
strong!' and I was getting really pissed off with him, shouting,
'No I can't!' and begging him to throw me out the window,
which made him laugh as the window was only about a foot
above ground level. Eventually, Julie tapped him on the shoulder, took him outside the room, and said: 'Really, she can't.
She needs the epidural.' I think he was actually a bit disappointed. He was absolutely convinced I would be able to get
through it on the power of my mind alone, and he was really
getting into the supporting role.

The anaesthetist put the needle into my spine, I had to stay
absolutely still through three contractions, which was very
hard. I had one arm around Tara's neck and one arm around
Julie's, to steady myself. To begin with, the epidural didn't take

the pain away, so they turned it up higher, and I went to sleep. I woke up an hour and a half later and I couldn't feel anything, so I asked them to turn it down. The doctor examined me and I was 7 cm dilated – a huge advance. Forty-five minutes later she measured me again and I was 10 cm! She was so amazed that she blurted out, 'Fuck girl, he's coming!' The epidural hadn't had time to wear off – I still couldn't feel anything from the waist down – so I had to watch the monitor to see when the contractions were coming to push. I was lying on my side with my eyes fixed on the monitor, and they were yelling at me to push as hard as I could. They said that I pushed better on an epidural than anyone they had ever seen!

Rafael's head was crowning and I put a hand on his head, and I remember feeling worried that it felt squooshy and it shouldn't feel that squooshy. The doctor had asked Cisco if he wanted to catch him and of course he did, but then she got worried that Rafael was looking grey so she just got him out as quickly as she could. They didn't tell me about that at the time, and fortunately he changed colour pretty quickly. I just hoped that he was all right. One of his eyes was open and one was closed, and I was worrying whether that eye was OK. He was already crying, which made me very happy when I heard it.

The first thing I did was to put him to my breast. There was a really happy intense feeling in the room, and a couple of friends of mine were right outside the door. They'd come to check on me and just happened to arrive at exactly the right time. I was tired, but I wasn't worn out. I felt great, I was really happy that the whole thing was over. If it had been up to me I could have gone home immediately, but my blood pressure didn't go down much so I was on medication. He was born at 9.54 p.m., and we went home at around 11 the next morning. He had a good night's sleep and he was in bed with me. The nursing [breastfeeding] got off to a pretty good start.

There wasn't much I would have changed, or had the power to change. I'd like not to have had high blood pressure, and then I wouldn't have had to be induced, so without pitocin the pain might not have been as intense and I might not have needed an epidural. Still, I'm really glad I had one; without it I'd probably have ended up with a C-section, and the thought of that terrified me. Looking back on it, I think I was *too* alternative about not wanting to have an epidural. The baby didn't come out dopey at all. It didn't even give me a backache. I was pissed off that they made me sit in a wheelchair to leave the hospital the next morning – I was fine!

N.B. One of the reasons why an epidural was given for Allegra's labour, to lower her blood pressure, can also make the procedure dangerous for a small percentage of women. At the Royal College of Midwives' annual conference in May 2004, midwives called for an urgent review of 'vastly overused' epidurals, which are now given to one in five women in UK hospitals, and as much as one in three in some areas. Said Claire Wood, a midwife for West London Hospital, 'The risks are rarely discussed with women in any detail and are often omitted from the discussion.' The most serious risk if an epidural goes wrong is a dramatic fall in blood pressure, which can be life-threatening for both mother and baby. Less dramatic risks include a greater likelihood of giving birth with the need for episiotomy, ventouse or forceps, and for the birth ending up as a Caesarean section.

18

Yoga Birth

Janet Balaskas is the founder of the Active Birth Centre in north London and a pioneer of antenatal yoga classes. In 1981 she organized a rally with 6,000 people, dubbed a 'squat in', to protest against the Royal Free Hospital's ban against women giving birth in upright positions. Janet has four children of her own, has had one orgasmic birth and one water birth, aged 42, and there is little doubt that her own wonderful birth experiences were the driving force behind helping women to achieve the same. Here, in much abbreviated form, she offers the edited highlights of all four of her births.

I had a pretty good first birth, but was given an unnecessary episiotomy [snip] that made me feel that I wanted to have my next baby at home. I had gone back to my native South Africa to have my first child in a small clinic where I was told I could have a natural birth. In between the birth of my first and second child I came back to live in England.

By the time I was pregnant with my second baby, I had become very keen on yoga and had trained with the

National Childbirth Trust (NCT) as a childbirth educator. What was going on in hospitals at the time [1976] was pretty horrific: there was a lot of routine high-tech management, so I decided that I wanted a home birth for my second. At that time there were only two independent midwives in London. They were called the Divine Light midwives, and I had one of them – Kate Russell. Having an independent midwife was the only way of planning an active birth at home at the time, and it was wonderful to know who the midwife was and to have a relationship with her throughout my pregnancy. At the same time I was researching birth to find out what happened during birth historically and in different cultures. As a result I understood the importance of being upright in labour, and I decided that I wanted to squat to give birth. By a stroke of luck, my NHS GP had been on holiday in Botswana and seen a woman squatting to give birth just before I was due, so it seemed like everything conspired to get the birth I wanted.

My midwife had never delivered in any position other than lying down; people just didn't know about anything other than semi-reclining in those days. But she said, 'I don't mind what position you are in.' My GP had asked specifically if he could come along, and he helped and encouraged me to squat. At the crucial moment, just when I felt like giving up, he reminded me that I wanted to give birth squatting and assisted me into the position. Once I was there it felt so much easier to push, and I managed to give birth without tearing, despite the fact that my daughter had an unusually large head. The midwife thought that squatting helped her to be born without assistance by opening the pelvic outlet to its maximum. I was thrilled and empowered by this experience.

My son and third child, Jed, was also born at home 20 months later, with the same midwife assisting me. This time, instead of squatting I was on all fours in the corridor between the bathroom and the bedroom! Jed weighed 10 lb 4 oz and yet, despite his size, this was the only birth I experienced that was completely painless – not a painless labour, but a painless birth. When people say that birth can be like an orgasm, this was a truly orgasmic birth. The whole birth, from the intense contractions at the end of labour to the expulsive stage, happened in under 3 minutes and I felt incredible afterwards – it was an amazing experience. I'm glad to have had one birth out of four like that. It was what Michel Odent [the pioneering French obstetrician who introduced water births in French public hospitals] calls 'the foetus ejection reflex' – when the birth happens involuntarily and very fast – what it could be like for many more women in the right circumstances. You need the right environment to produce a high level of hormones for that to happen, and this birth was a very private, personal and quiet experience with only my husband assisting. Even the midwife stayed mostly in the background and left us alone. I felt I needed my partner there for emotional support, it was very important he was there – he made me feel safe.

I was at 6 cm dilation. The midwife had just examined me, so I thought, 'I've got a way to go, I'll have a bath.' My husband was sitting behind the door while I was in the bathroom. I put my foot in the water and I thought suddenly that getting into the bath was a bad idea, I had to be on the floor on my hands and knees instead. I thought I was going to be sick. I remember having this thought, thinking 'What's he [my husband] going to think about me, this is going to put him off for ever' and then he said 'Just let go, that's great!' I did let go at that moment, and seconds later my son was being born. My husband said, 'It's a boy and his eyes are open' when only his head was born – then his body came out and as he was passed to me between my legs I saw that he was right!

My fourth child, Theo, was born at home 10 years later. I decided I wanted the obstetrician Michel Odent there, as the Divine Light midwives were no longer practising. I wanted to try out Michel Odent's foetus ejection reflex theory – I'd pretty much had one before with my previous birth – and also Michel's belief in privacy in labour. This meant I would be on my own during much of it, with Michel very much present but in the background.

Theo was unusually big, born at around 11 lb; I was huge at the end of that pregnancy. Because I was 42 years old, I had my check-ups with Yehudi Gordon [the obstetrician at St John's and Elizabeth's Hospital in London, and author of *Birth and Beyond*, published recently by Vermilion] and everything was fine. Three years previously I had an operation to remove a uterine fibroid, but nevertheless Yehudi gave his approval for a home birth. I also had a scan at 14 weeks, and was in a dilemma over whether to have an amniocentesis [an invasive test where a thin needle is inserted into the amniotic sac and amniotic fluid is drawn out for chromosomal analysis]. When I saw the scan I had a strong feeling that the baby was fine, and this was confirmed while sitting in quiet meditation a few days later. That is one of the things that can happen in yoga – you have a clearer unconscious connection with your baby and a deeper inner guidance that can help you to make important decisions.

This time I had a waterbirth pool to use for relaxation and pain-relief during labour, but because of the size of the baby, Michel wasn't keen that I give birth in water. The labour was incredibly intense and I was so uncomfortable before I got in the pool – no position seemed to relieve the pain. Getting into the water made an enormous difference to how I felt – the increase in comfort was dramatic. Suddenly even squatting was easy and comfortable, and it was bliss to relax in between the contractions. Apparently three hours of labour had gone by when Michel said that it was time to come out of the pool. I protested, saying 'but I've only just got in,' and he told me it was time to make a change. I had no idea how long I had been in the pool. Michel examined me in the pool and could see that I was ready; people are often ready when they mention the word 'death' and I had said that I felt like I was going to 'drown or die in the pool'. I got out and was standing up with my husband behind me when, seven contractions later, still standing, Michel caught the baby at my feet. He handed me Theo, saying 'Here is your big boy.' There was no tearing. After the first episiotomy, I never tore with the subsequent three births. I think that has to do with the environment, because I birthed them at home, in privacy. I felt very comfortable and my body could relax.

I've practised yoga through three of my pregnancies, and I've never needed any pain-relief at all. I put the rising C-section rate today down to the overuse of induction and epidurals in hospitals. If people were able to incorporate some of the principles of an active birth into such medical situations, it would help to prevent foetal distress, relax the mother and reduce the rate of Caesareans. Essentially a change of consciousness is needed, so that birth is perceived as hormonal, sexual and emotional, rather than a medical experience. It is only medical when intervention is needed – and hospital is not a place to go to have a sexual experience.

Janet's Principles of Yoga and Active Birth

I started teaching Active Birth in the 1970s, and one of my main criticisms of childbirth education at that time was that it mostly revolved around talk and lectures, held in the last weeks of pregnancy. This sort of preparation is very cerebral and limited. It only appeals to the thinking mind of a pregnant woman – probably the least important part while giving birth – and nothing was offered to help prepare the body for giving birth. I noticed from researching birth in other cultures that many yoga positions resembled the natural upright positions for birth, and it occurred to me that practising yoga might be a very good way to prepare for birth. You have nine months to get yourself ready. A pregnant woman's body changes to accommodate her baby, and so does her consciousness – physically, emotionally, psychologically and spiritually. Yoga works along with the natural process happening in a woman's body, encouraging the release of the hormones that trigger and promote the birth process. It teaches you to release tension and to relax – to trust your body to do its work.

It also takes a woman on a journey within herself, which is where she is going to have to go when in labour. It quiets the mind and makes the way free for unthinking, instinctual behaviour. Often our minds are cluttered with thought, there is a lot of stimulus to the intellectual part of the brain – the neo-cortex – which becomes dormant during labour. The back of the brain, however, called the 'old brain' where the pituitary gland lies, is very active in labour, producing hormones such as oxytocin – and this is the part of a woman you want to appeal to. So yoga is relaxing and calming, it helps the woman to develop the ability to focus her awareness inside herself, to shut the world out, and is meditational exercise. There are many different forms of yoga, many of which are focused mainly on achieving postures, whereas the type of yoga I practise is both strong and gentle and its power lies more in the focus on breathing and gravity. This was developed from classical Hatha Yoga and adapted specifically for pregnancy. By now we have the evidence of more than 25 years of experience to know that this way of preparing for birth and motherhood is very effective.

Unlike many yoga positions, nothing that we do is likely to be difficult. If a posture or a movement feels uncomfortable we have pillows to make it more comfortable, and generally it's fine for women to leave it out – unless it is specifically designed to help women maintain concentration during a contraction. For example, we practise a standing squat that works the thigh muscles and challenges you to stay in one position and keep breathing through the discomfort, like breathing through the pain of a contraction. Going through birth is a huge and challenging experience. Just like a mountaineer facing the challenge of climbing Everest – you wouldn't want to do that unprepared.

It's best to join a pregnancy yoga class at around four months of pregnancy and to make the most of the remaining months. Today, however, I had a call from a woman who came to just three yoga classes right at the end of her pregnancy and, even so, had a wonderful birth. Somehow she got exactly what she needed. My goal generally is to inspire women to have the confidence that they can do this; they can get through the pain of contractions, surrender to the process and let the body take over. Birth is beyond our conscious control – the art is to relax, let go, lose one's inhibitions and let it happen.

Janet Balaskas' latest book, *The Waterbirth Book*, is published by Thorsons.

19

Caesarean Birth

There are lots of good reasons why you might have to have a Caesarean. For all the mud-slinging that goes on between doctors and midwives, mothers and the media on the subject, the fact remains that C-sections still account for 21.5 per cent of all births in the UK. That means that two out of the ten people sitting in your antenatal class may end up having one.

In April 2004, the National Institute of Clinical Excellence published their findings on Caesareans, after years of research. One of the more surprising titbits in the report was evidence suggesting that 'having another woman with you for support during labour reduces the risk of Caesarean section.' Among all the risks and statistics, this nugget offers a human face on all the medical facts: that just by having a familiar friend with you, as well as your partner, you might escape the knife. It is a reminder that birth is not only a physical process, something highlighted in Kate Houston's Caesarean birth story below, but also an emotional one, too.

To prepare mentally for a C-section, **first the word 'failure' must be banned from your vocabulary**. It enters your head the moment a doctor sticks the label 'failure to progress' on your notes as a reason to move to theatre. The NCT are campaigning on behalf of all women to have the phrase 'failure to progress' changed to something less damaging to the female psyche. The psychologist Joan Raphael Leff maintains that it is not uncommon for a woman who has given birth by Caesarean 'to feel so guilt-ridden at having deprived her baby of birth-canal stimulation and spontaneous birth that she may believe she has predetermined her/his personality to bypass conflict, avoid work and/or seek premature gratification'.[1] Motherhood is not a race, and if you don't have a normal birth you haven't fallen at the first hurdle. In the greater spiritual scheme of things, whatever happens to you and your baby is the right lesson for you both to learn at that time. And research has shown that it is better for babies to experience some labour before being born by Caesarean than none at all.[2]

Once you know that you are having a C-section, gather as much help as you can around you for the postnatal period. You are going to have to adapt to motherhood in the hardest possible way, after a major operation, and you will need others to fetch, carry and mother you afterwards. Ask the doctor to explain this to your partner, before leaving the hospital. All too often husbands expect their wives to be back to normal when they look well. Even if you feel pretty chipper after the birth, buoyed up by those birth hormones, you will still need to take things easy to prevent a post-operative slump, or the risk of the scar opening. I have two friends who took on too much at the beginning of their recovery period, and both had to return to hospital with complications as a result. A survey done by Dr Charles Wolfe of the Department of Public Health Medicine interviewed 49,000 women in the southeast and found that 65 per cent of women had not recovered after three months and reported problems with tiredness, backache or depression. You want to be part of the other 35 per cent.

Finally, take something for the shock to the system. The Bach Flower treatment Rescue Remedy can be swigged during and afterwards for as long as you replay the mental video of the birth in your mind. Kate Figes, author of *Life After Birth*, found a trip to the homoeopath helpful after her second Caesarean:

I went to see a homoeopath because I just didn't feel well, and as I recounted my experience of childbirth I burst into tears, for it felt so real, as if it had happened yesterday. She [the homoeopath] could tell that I was still in a state of shock and believed that the morphine I had been given through the epidural had frozen the shock moments after birth in a sort of time warp. She gave me homoeopathic opium and within days, I felt much better. The memories of childbirth began to fade and the scar healed quickly.

Emergency C-section

Kate Houston, a world-championship medallist in the Modern Pentathlon, was 33 when she gave birth to her daughter Cordelia by Caesarean section. Kate's labour was progressing well, but slowed temporarily when she went into hospital. They broke her waters in hospital and gave her an epidural, after which there were concerns about the baby's heart rate, so she was advised to have an emergency C-section. After the birth she moved from the hospital to a birth centre, which turned a difficult experience into a positive one.

During my pregnancy I had the option of a midwife-run birthing centre called Wallingford Cottage Hospital or the John Radcliffe Hospital in Oxford. I was assuming, as most first-time mothers do, that I was going to be late, so when I went into labour on my due date and my midwife was away that weekend, I was a bit taken by surprise.

On Saturday I had had a 'show' when the mucus plug came out around midday. But there were no contractions and I didn't think much about it, so I went off to see a horse that afternoon, and was the proud owner of 'Elvis' on my return. I came home and my waters broke at 10 p.m. on Saturday night. My first reaction was shock, and I phoned the Wallingford Cottage Hospital and told them my waters had broken and there were no contractions. At that point I still hadn't made up my mind whether to go for the midwives at the Wallingford or the John Radcliffe Hospital. The midwife on duty at the Wallingford said, 'If you're not convinced, go to the JR.'

So we went into the JR, there were still no contractions, and they examined me on arrival. I was 1-2 cm dilated and not in full-blown labour, so they said, 'Go home and rest, but come back within 24 hours.' I went home, got some sleep (there were only a few contractions), but as I was restless I got up and finished off my expenses and emails, and at 5a.m. went off to feed the horses. When my husband Dominic got up we went for a long four-hour walk (as I thought this was meant to get labour going) and a pub lunch (I didn't feel like eating much, though).

We went home and I was going to rest in the bath for a while when my brother and his girlfriend suddenly showed up for tea. When they'd left I went up for a lie-down, at which point I noticed that the contractions had got stronger and more regular, around 5 minutes apart. Our 24 hours were up, so we went into the JR and were attended by a midwife who had been on duty all night. She said, 'You're 3-4 cm dilated, so you can go home.' At that moment I lost confidence in her – after all, we had come back in after 24 hours because we had been told to. She left the room, and my labour had pretty much shut down, so I said to Dom that I didn't have confidence in the midwife and didn't understand what was going on, but Dom told me not to make a fuss. When she came back in the room and said, 'Yes, you're right, you are supposed to stay in, we will move you to a delivery room,' I felt by then that I was just waiting for the shift to change so she would go off-duty. We tried to get things going again by (yet more) walking up and down the hospital corridors – trying to avoid the busy-looking uniforms ...

The new midwife who came along was excellent, she explained that she thought my hind-waters had broken but not my fore-waters, and she suggested rupturing the membranes as a form of induction. As soon as she did this, the contractions set off with a vengeance. When I sat down, however, I noticed that both my legs were shaking, something that only happened when I was totally exhausted after doing a hard circuit session in training. I also felt quite cold, something that also happens to my body when I am exhausted after a tough bout of running and riding. I noted this to myself, but didn't mention it to anyone else. It was then that I asked for pain-relief and was given some gas and air, and I used it like a scuba diver, visualizing coral under the sea with my eyes shut, which worked really well. However, with the gas and air, and contractions coming so fast, I wasn't very mobile.

By this time, my darling husband Dom had eaten all my food and was lying on the floor of the delivery suite with a pillow under his head snoring away! I left him asleep and the midwife and I had a good laugh, and I asked her how long she thought I might have to go. She said 'Probably six or seven hours' and my heart sank. I think if she had said to me, 'You're doing really well, why don't we change positions?' or something like that I would have felt differently, but instead I asked for more pain-relief as I didn't think I could cope.

She offered Meptid, which is a less strong form of pethidine, mentioning that it would send me a bit 'out of it', or an epidural. A good friend of mine had had a good birth experience with an epidural, so I went with the epidural, which was organized quickly and was put in between contractions. The epidural, however, just immobilized me further, and even with a top-up it wasn't working in the stomach area where it was needed. Apparently, in 15 per cent of cases epidurals don't work, and I was one of those statistics. I think because I am 5 ft 11in and everyone gets the same dose I should have been given a man's quantity to anaesthetize the area. So it was back to the gas and air, with even less mobility.

With the epidural they put a trace on the baby (routine policy), which resulted in concern about the baby's heartbeat. The senior midwife came in to look at the trace and we began to get into an escalating process of intervention. When Dominic woke up I felt a bit sorry for him because he'd gone to sleep and everything had been fine, and he woke up and all this intervention had started. They got an obstetrician in and he wanted to take blood samples from the baby's scalp. I was only comfortable lying on my right-hand side and they wanted me to lie on the left, and then there were four people in the room – obstetrician, senior midwife, midwife and nurse.

My contractions were still going strong, they took a sample but the blood clotted on the way to the lab, so they had to come back and try again. Again it clotted, and each time I had to lie still while they pushed a 12-inch glass needle up me to get the sample from the baby's head. The blood sample was to get an oxygen reading, but after three attempts they had to abandon the idea.

Then they offered to leave us for 40 minutes. And when they came in to check, they were concerned that the baby's heart rate wasn't responding well to the contractions, there wasn't much explanation, just that it was 'dipping in and out with not enough variation', and they said that possibly the baby was asleep (because the heart rate slows down then) or there was a problem. By now they had also picked up a slight placental tear and they were concerned that the tear could be a sign of a bigger abruption to come, and they wanted the baby out within an hour.

The doctor then did an internal examination to see how dilated I was and said I was 7 cm. He said that there was no way I was going to get to 10 cm in an hour, so he wanted to move to a C-section. I asked for more time, 'Couldn't we have another hour?', but he answered, 'You risk cerebral palsy or brain damage, etc'. As soon as he said that I said, 'Fine, wheel me up there now.' I turned to Dom, who was looking a little green, and told him that he didn't have to come with me as I was fine. It was about 3 a.m. by now, and I had had the epidural around 1 a.m., so it all seemed to be happening incredibly fast. It was so confusing.

Because the epidural hadn't worked, they needed to give a spinal block on top of the epidural and then asked me whether I could feel my legs. I answered 'Yes.' Then, using this amazing electronic bed I was on, they jiggled and shook me around a bit and after a top-up I was numb. Then I was looking around the room a bit, ignoring my bottom half, when this good-looking surgeon walks into the theatre all dressed up in his scrubs and I remember thinking 'Phwoar, I fancy him!', until I looked again and realized it was Dom, whom I hadn't expected to see! He came over and stood by my head.

I didn't feel a thing through the whole procedure. I know some people say that it is like doing the dishes in your stomach or rummaging in a handbag, but I had none of that sensation. When they pulled her out, she was tinged a little blue and they said 'baby girl' and then rushed her over to the other side of the room to resuscitate her – nobody said anything, and it was the longest minute ever. Then I heard her yell and there was great relief. They asked if Dom wanted to weigh the baby and asked us to guess the weight, I said '9 lb 2oz' and she was 9 lb 1¾ oz.

All the staff in theatre were very kind and nice throughout. They put her on me, and Dom held her while they sewed me up. I think when Dom went to weigh her, he peered over the screen and saw all my innards and was a little traumatized by that. Cordi was born at 3.30 a.m., and by 6.30 a.m. Dom had left the hospital to get some sleep and go on to a board meeting, but I think he was in shock and didn't know what to do.

Looking back on it, I was very lucky. I had no infections, backache or tiredness and was able to transfer to the Wallingford

Cottage Hospital the next day, which turned the whole experience round for me. I had lots of attention, support and peace, unlike in a major teaching hospital where midwives are rushed off their feet. Looking back on the birth, I had assumed that birth was a physical process and therefore – being a very physically fit sort of person – that I'd be able to do it and I would be fine. But I had neglected the psychological and emotional side, and was not that well prepared despite those NCT classes. I hadn't appreciated the psychological and emotional aspect of birth (which is probably 90 per cent), because everyone says birth is physical.

The Wallingford midwives were amazing, supportive emotionally and practically, changing my birth from a traumatic one to a positive one. The food there was good (healthy salads and plenty of carbohydrates and homemade cakes) and they had time to talk to me, to show me how to rub vitamin E into the scar to help it heal, and encouraged me to look at my scar and feel it (unlike another friend, who was too scared to touch hers for a year). They also recommended arnica for bruising (i.e. surgery) and tea tree oil for the bath (as a natural antiseptic to avoid infection), both of which helped get me back on my feet. They also really helped me to get breastfeeding going (which was a natural healer, having had such an interventionist birth), by giving me their time.

(Kate learned a lesson from her first birth, particularly how she reacted mentally and emotionally to the hospital set-up, and went on to have a triumphant second birth at home, birthing little Olivia Athenae on her bathroom floor in one magnificent push. I felt honoured to be there.)

The National Institute of Clinical Excellence (NICE) guidelines for Caesarean sections were published in April 2004, and a version for women can be downloaded free from the NICE website: www.nice.org.uk. A more detailed discussion of the individual recommendations can also be obtained from www.caesarean.org.uk

20

Vaginal Birth After Caesarean (VBAC)

Jenny Lesley, from Worthing in West Sussex, had three Caesarean sections before getting the birth she wanted, a gentle birth at home in a pool, aged 39.

Jenny was 28 when she was given her first emergency Caesarean during labour. She had been in pre-labour for 24 hours before they broke her waters, on the Saturday night before Christmas. On her notes were written 'failure to progress', but she was told in labour that her baby 'was in distress'. Studying her notes later, she saw that the baby's apgar score was 9 out of a maximum of 10, showing her newborn to be pink, alert and with good reflexes – no distress recorded.

With her second baby, she was labelled 'high risk' because of the previous Caesarean. She was told to go in early, at the first contraction, to her local hospital Southlands, near Worthing, and after her waters broke, according to hospital protocol, she was induced within 24 hours. This started an 'intervention cascade' as she remembers, with an epidural to cope with the strength of the contractions after induction, then problems pushing out the baby with an anaesthetized lower half, a ventouse that didn't work and finally another Caesarean section. During her second section, Jenny spent four hours in the operating theatre because she had lost so much blood that they thought her bladder might have been 'nicked' by the surgeon's knife. She needed a blood transfusion as a result, but 'mercifully I escaped infections and had no problems conceiving again'.

By the third birth, I had trained as an antenatal teacher and was determined that my body could have done it in both cases if my labour had been managed better. This time I had booked in Crawley Hospital and was living in East Grinstead. I had persuaded the head of midwifery and consultant obstetrician to try for a VBAC if I went into labour spontaneously. At my 40-week routine appointment, my blood pressure was high and I had protein in the urine – suspected pre-eclampsia. It is highly unusual for a third-time mother to develop pre-eclampsia, and now I was faced with this scenario that I could either wait to go into labour or wait to go into a fit. Although the third section was classed as an emergency, it was a reasonably calm and positive experience, and I was sitting up and breastfeeding soon after, but there was still this slight niggle that I hadn't needed it, my blood pressure always seemed to be particularly high on the ward.

But it was the psychological and emotional impact of the three sections that had hit Jenny the hardest later. 'I was depressed after the first C-section. I felt incredibly worthless, had mood swings and low self-esteem because I felt that I had failed to give birth and wasn't able to breastfeed. My body had not functioned as I expected, and I felt the label of "failure to progress" hard to live with.' This depression went on for months and Jenny went back to work early, after 12 weeks, suffering terrible recurrent migraines. 'Postnatal depression felt like another failure,' says Jenny 'I had failed to give birth, breastfeed and now I had PND [postnatal depression]. My poor husband had to bear with me sobbing in the night in the middle of the bed.'

There was a five-year gap between the third and the fourth baby. Jenny had been working as an antenatal teacher and read a lot of research about supporting women during labour. 'When I watched the little blue line appear, I thought "I'm not having a Caesar." I was determined to give my body the chance to do what I felt it could do and knew that birth could be a wonderful, uplifting experience rather than an awful and painful one.'

Her first move was to hire independent midwives to support her through the experience of labour and birth. True to form with her previous labours, she went overdue, this time by as much as 11 days (or possibly 18 days, depending on how the dates were calculated) and was longing to give birth by the time labour started.

I spent a restless night, not unusual for me, getting up to the loo every hour or so, and aware that I had reasonably constant period pain, but not daring to hope it was significant after so many previous 'is this it?' moments. At half-past six I decided it was officially morning and got up to use the loo and perhaps have a bath. I realized as I went to the loo that I was having a strong twinge/contraction, and had another one on the way back. My first thought was that these could be Braxton Hicks, as they were too close together to be early labour contractions. I pottered around the bedroom having more every 5 minutes, and told my husband Raymond that I didn't think he should go to work as this might be it. But I still didn't really believe it even though I knew the pains were really contractions now.

We got the kids up and started the getting-them-ready-for-school/breakfast/lunch-boxes nightmare that is a Monday morning in our house. I had to keep ducking behind the fridge freezer to breathe through the pains, which were holding at 5 minutes apart and needed concentration to deal with. I had a bowl of cereal in the sitting room while Ray did the lunch-boxes and I decided to phone my midwife Mary Cronk to let her know what was happening. I didn't expect her to come out to me, I was officially Andrya Prescott's responsibility now as Mary was due to go to a conference on the 1 p.m. train, but I wanted her to know that I was in labour, because she had been my main midwife all the way through. After that I rang Andrya and she said she would aim to be with me with her support midwife, Sue, about 10.30 a.m.

Mary rang me again about 8 a.m. offering to pop in on her way to the conference. I was starting to get concerned that things were hotting up a bit, but still couldn't believe we were looking at a quick labour. My concern was only could I stand up to 12 hours plus of this!

By the time Raymond left to take the kids to school I was over the birthing ball and feeling a bit panicky about being on my own for half an hour, so Raymond stopped off at my friend Lesley's house and she came over to be with me until Ray got back just after 9a.m.

I got Ray to time how long the contractions were lasting as they seemed longer. They were lasting a minute and coming every 4 to 5 minutes. I was saying 'oooooooh', which seemed to be my way of breathing through the contractions until Mary arrived at 9.55 a.m. and I was so happy to see her. Having sadly accepted that I was not going to be able to have her at the birth, it was a real treat to see her familiar face.

Meanwhile the contractions carried on inexorably and I discovered that walking about between them, and then holding on to the mantelpiece while Raymond rubbed my back, was the best way of dealing with them.

Andrya and Sue arrived at 10.30 a.m.: I had met Andrya once before, but Sue was a new face and I felt a bit shy initially. Mary, I think sensing this, offered to cancel her Brighton visit and stay on as long as she could. Andrya asked me whether I would like a VE [vaginal examination] to assess progress. By this time I was desperate to know was this really it and was my cervix dilating, so we went upstairs. I was worried about having to lie down for a VE – I couldn't see how anyone could possibly labour lying down, I needed to be up, up, up. I hung on to the door, mimicking the NCT birth-positions poster for a contraction, while Andrya got ready, then lunged for the bed at the last possible minute. Andrya was gentle and quick and gave me the best news ever: at least 3-4 cm dilated and effacing well [as well as the cervix dilating, it also thins out and becomes more stretchy – known as 'effacing']. Wow! I had been dreading her saying 'Oh, only 1 cm,' and was delighted that I had gain in return for the pain.

By 11.10 I was wondering about getting into the pool – I was concerned it might be too early and would slow things down. I was still convinced that I had hours and hours of this to go, and asked Raymond to make arrangements for his mum to pick up the children from school and take them to her house overnight. I decided to get in the pool, encouraged by Andrya and Sue, who were pottering about getting their equipment set up. Mary was calculating how late she could leave it and still catch her train!

The pool was like a welcoming old friend giving you a hug. I had used it so much during the wait for labour that it was a familiar, safe place, somewhere I associated with relief from aches and pains. I half-knelt, half-floated, arms and elbows on the side. Sue was near me, asking me if it helped, Raymond was issuing his mum with sleeping bags for the children in the other room. As I 'aaahed' and 'oohed' my way through a contraction, I hoped briefly that my mother-in-law wasn't too embarrassed.

By 11.30 things were starting to really hurt. Mary gave me some coaching to encourage me to keep breathing through the pain: 'Try to go saggy with it,' I remember her saying.

By midday (I only know timings because of the midwives' record), I was at the 'I don't want to give birth anymore!' stage. I wondered if I was in transition, and I wondered how I could possibly survive this pain. From all round the room voices of encouragement came. 'Yes you can do this, you *are* doing this, you are fantastic, you are strong.' Ray was by my head all the time, breathing with me, soothing me, putting a hand on my back. I got enormous solace just from his presence, and by rubbing my face up and down his forearm like a cat!

I started to feel an urge to push but it was all mixed up with the awful, overwhelming last contractions of 'first stage'. I invoked my Maker a lot to get me through those. And throughout I had a really strong sense of the Lord being with me and of being surrounded by His love. I think Mary had left by then, but I could still hear her voice telling me I could do this, mixed with Andrya and Sue telling me the same thing. The mixture of female empathy and male strength was just amazing, I never really felt alone and I certainly felt that both Andrya and Sue knew just how I was feeling. I was on hands and knees in the pool through all this, rocking backwards and forwards through each rollercoaster contraction, alternating out-breaths with moaning, but mostly feeling I had control. There were a couple of really scary contractions where I felt they were winning and I was losing it, really crying out in panic. The voices soothed me and I began to find that pushing made the pain better.

I was not altogether sure what I should be pushing where. I did have a sense of the baby but was actually more aware of a need to poo. At 12.35 Andrya records me saying 'Oh, Andrya, the baby moved' and it was a real revelation to feel this solid football thing actually shifting inside me, getting closer. I can remember thinking 'I'm actually going to do this' and saying 'Yes, yes, yes' with the pushes.

I heard myself begin to bellow and thought, 'This really does mean not long now,' remembering that you only get a few like that before the baby arrives. Andrya asked me a couple of times did I want to feel what was happening, but by now I had stretched myself horizontally across the pool, hands pushing my head away from the side, legs apart but pushing from the other side. It worked wonderfully. I could feel all my effort paying off, and kept bearing down and letting the air out, grunting and breathing out, swallowing the occasional bit of water when I forgot to keep my head up!

I started to feel stinging down there. 'Bl**dy hell' was all I could think, 'I've talked about this so much in classes and now it's happening to ME!' 'Blow, blow, blow' Andrya was telling me. I was keen to listen to her, I desperately didn't want to tear. I blew for England and it really didn't hurt as much as I had expected it to, as his head emerged. I was aware of Andrya helping the baby a little – she explained afterwards that his hips were a bit stuck and there was lots of meconium [the baby's poo] in the water. I didn't care, it felt like a good thing.

He slithered out and she passed him through my legs to me and I managed to sit back and take my little boy. He looked a bit green and pale, and wasn't breathing, but his cord was pulsing. I just couldn't believe it. Ray came round to lean over and help keep the baby's head out of the water while I supported his body. I checked he really was a boy like the scan had said. 'Hello, little man,' I remember saying over and over, together with 'We DID it!'

Baby Fergus gradually established his breathing and the cord stopped pulsing. Andrya showed Raymond what to do and he cut the cord almost exactly as I felt a contraction and pushed the placenta out into the pool. The pool was now so murky that Andrya and I had to go fishing for it! Raymond took Fergus while I got gingerly out of the pool and sat on a pile of covered cushions and pillows on the floor. I was intact perineally, and it felt great. He was born at 12.50, weighing 8 lb 6 oz, and by 13.25 he was on the breast and I had a cheese and cucumber sandwich and a very welcome cup of tea. We sat for quite a while, talking in wonder about how quick and how powerful it had all been.

The children came back from school, shooting through the door like little bullets, desperate to see the new arrival. They

were completely thrilled by him and by the presents he had
'brought' them. By 10 o'clock we were all in bed, Fergus having defied all my usual predictions on baby behaviour after
feeding most of the evening.

For more information about going for a VBAC, see the
Association for Improvements in the Maternity Services
(AIMS) booklet on VBAC (written by Jenny Lesley
and published in 2004, price £5.50, p&p included, see
www.aims.org.uk). It gives you the facts to ponder on
about the risks of a C-section and repeat C-sections, the
low risk of scar rupture and the heartening statistic that
70 per cent of women who go for a VBAC, achieve it.
It highlights that a VBAC will enable faster recovery
time, less risk of infection/haemorrhage and future
complications. Also worth visiting is www.vbac.org.uk
for lots of birth stories and up-to-date statistics.

21

Helping Hands: Useful Contacts

If you need extra help to get the birth you want, or more information to make the right decision, call in the professionals:

Association for Improvements in the Maternity Services (AIMS)
(tel: 0870 765 1433)
www.aims.org.uk
AIMS has been offering support and advice to mothers in their birth choices for the past 40 years. It also has dozens of publications on everything from ultrasound to induction.

Independent Midwives Association (IMA)
1 The Great Quarry, Guildford, GU1 3XL (tel: 01483 821104)
www.independentmidwives.org.uk
The cost of hiring an independent midwife to assist you for antenatal visits, the labour and birth, and the postnatal period is around £2,500. Independent midwives will take on high-risk cases and in some cases

may be able to accompany you into your local hospital.

Association of Radical Midwives (ARM)
(tel: 0121 444 2257/helpline 01243 671673)
www.radmid.demon.co.uk
Support for women (and midwives) that are having difficulty in getting or giving appropriate midwifery care.

www.birthchoiceuk.com
All women are allowed to choose or change their
hospital at whatever point in their pregnancy, and this
website offers a list of questions to help you decide
what sort of care you want, and then matches the
answers to your local maternity unit.

National Childbirth Trust (NCT)
(tel: 0870 444 8707)
www.nctpregnancyandbabycare.com
An independent charity running antenatal classes,
breastfeeding counselling and postnatal support
network (with an irritating answerphone service and
confusing website).

Caroline Flint Midwifery Services
(tel: 020 7820 6661)
www.birthcentre.com
The past president of the Royal College of Midwives
Caroline Flint runs the only private birth centre in the
country, situated in South West London. The New
Family package costs £4,925.

Active Birth Centre
25 Bickerton Road
London N19 5JT
(tel: 020 7281 6760)
www.activebirthcentre.com
No births take place at the Active Birth Centre, but
there is plenty of information and mail order items,
therapy sessions and pool hire – as well as yoga classes
with Janet Balaskas.

Antenatal Results and Choices (ARC)
73 Charlotte Street, London W1 4PN
(tel: 020 7631 0285 helpline)
www.arc-uk.org.
Helps mothers and families understand results of antenatal tests and offers non-directive support.

Caesarean Support Network
(tel: 01624 661269 from 6pm to 9pm daily)
Support, information and counselling offered from a
service now running for 14 years.

Homebirth.org.uk
The mother Angela Horn has compiled comprehensive
information on home birth coupled with inspirational
birth stories on this excellent site.

THIRD STAGE

EIGHT WEEKS
TO GO

Where Do I Want to Give Birth?

You may feel it is a bit late in the day to answer this question, but the wonderful thing about being a Lady with an all-important Baby is that you have the power to change your mind about your birth right up to the day of labour. Ideally you should be able to revisit the decision in late pregnancy anyway, and be quite within your rights to change your mind without even justifying or explaining your decision. For example, in some areas of the country, such as Torbay, the community midwives do not book women anywhere, **they leave the decision about where to give birth open until the woman is in labour – then the mother decides where she would prefer to be**. As a result they have one of the highest home-birth rates and lowest intervention figures in the country.

When my hospital consultant explained at my 32-week appointment that 'we consider "term" for twins to be 36 weeks' and that I would be delivering in theatre with a dozen people present, I decided that that wasn't the scenario I had envisioned. I had just stopped work and hadn't really thought about the birth until then. After a couple of weeks researching a different alternative, I finally hired my independent midwives and opted for a home birth in my 34th week.

If any of the birth stories that you have read in the Second Stage have resonated with you, and you feel that you would like go for something a little beyond standard hospital fare, then now is the time to make that change. Most hospitals allow pregnant women to carry their notes with them, so while there may be surprise at your decision, or coercion to do otherwise, you can always gather up your notes and go elsewhere.

These are your options:

You Could Give Birth in Hospital Under Consultant-led Care

This 'medical model' of care might suit you if you would feel more comfortable being monitored closely, and aren't sure how much you'll be able to relax and trust your body or instincts. The 'medical model' of birth describes the attitude that childbirth should be seen as a risky event, safe only in retrospect. If there is some 'high-risk' element to your pregnancy, you may be told this is your 'only' option (which it isn't). See Birthchoice.co.uk for information about different maternity units in the UK and their statistics for use of intervention and Caesarean rates.

You Could Give Birth in Hospital under Midwifery-led Care

This 'midwifery model' of care will still use continuous monitoring during pregnancy and birth, but the midwives are more likely to seek and listen to the woman's views and to believe that childbirth is safe and that women's bodies are perfectly designed for it. If you opt for midwifery-led care, write a birth plan to discuss it in advance with your hospital and community midwives to see what will and won't be encouraged on the day.

You Could Give Birth in a Birth Centre under Midwifery-led Care

If you have an NHS Birth Centre nearby, and are deemed a low-risk pregnancy, you may feel this is an alternative to a hospital birth. Birth Centres are very much more accountable to the individual than a hospital, where you are treated as if you have walked in off the street (which you have). 'Birth centres provide a focus for midwives, a safe haven for the practice of "real midwifery", a place where like-minded midwives can turn the rhetoric of modern maternity care into reality ...' writes Mavis Kirkham in the book *Birth Centres: A Social Model for Maternity Care* (Books for Midwives, an imprint of Elsevier). If you are lucky enough to have a local Birth Centre, visit it first to meet the midwives and to see whether you like the atmosphere.

You Could Give Birth at Home on the NHS

Every woman in this country has a right to a home birth *whatever her level of risk*, under the Government's Changing Childbirth manifesto in 1993, which is still official policy. If you are finding any kind of resistance to this option, which is frequently the case, make sure that the real reason is not lack of midwives or expertise rather than some overt or covert suggestion about your suitability. Don't be fobbed off with 'most first-time mothers transfer' or any other excuse. Home birth doesn't suit NHS Trusts because it requires two midwives to be present (as opposed to one midwife looking after four women in hospital) which mucks up their rotas. If all else fails and you are wedded to the idea, call Beverley Beech at the Association for Improvements in the Maternity Services (AIMS, tel. 0870 765 1433) who will help support your cause.

You Could Give Birth at Home with Independent Midwives

Independent midwives can only birth you at home, although a few do have special relationships with doctors within hospitals if you want them to accompany you into hospital. The independent midwife can be taken on at any time up to the birth, although many will be booked beforehand or prefer to take you on earlier, and will take care of your antenatal and postnatal care. They cost around £2,500 at the time of writing, and are usually skilled and experienced, providing that continuous care and familiar face that most mothers crave. There are no independent midwives in Northern Ireland and few in Scotland and Wales, although some will travel. (See section on independent midwives in Can You Feel It?, page 88.)

You Could Give Birth in a Private Hospital

All the private hospitals are in London, which is a pain if you live in Dumfries. However, should your insurance cover it or you want to birth in style with a candle-lit champagne supper after delivery, you will be guaranteed hot-and-cold running staff to pamper you. The consultants and midwives may be no more qualified than their NHS counterparts, however. Some, such as the celebs' favourite The Portland Hospital, have midwife-led care as well as consultant-led care, and so are not just for the too-smart-to-stretch crowd. Others include St John and St Elizabeth for great waterbirth facilities, the Lindo Wing of St Mary's, and private areas within Chelsea & Westminster and Queen Charlotte's. Expect to pay around £3,500 for the consultant's charge, £350 for the anaesthetist's charge for an epidural, plus around £1,200 for your first 24 hours' care with scans and consultant paediatricians as extra.

You Could Give Birth in a Private Birth Centre

There is only one truly private Birth Centre and that is in southwest London and run by the indomitable Caroline Flint, past president of the Royal College of Midwives, who has a keen and experienced team under her wing. The brochure (with its 'As Seen in *Vogue*' sticker) paints an alternative and more gentle view of how your birth could go. Costs start from around £3,725, depending on where you pick up the care. Tel: 020 7820 6661 or visit www.birthcentre.com.

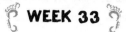

WEEK 33

Antenatal Classes

Your antenatal classes should have started by now, and if they haven't and you want to attend, sign up. Generally speaking there are two sorts of antenatal classes – those organized by the hospital and those offered by the NCT or an Active Birth Centre. Most will have been booked by women about three months into their pregnancy, although sometimes there are drop-outs or a waiting list is set up, so it's never too late to ask.

As Pat Thomas says in *Your Birth Rights* (The Women's Press, 2002), 'Antenatal classes are ideally placed to support women and help them feel powerful and important during this time. Unfortunately, they instead tend to provide persuasive advertising for a "sensible" hospital birth with all the benefits of technology and the many different gadgets that can be used to "get" the baby out.'

This was certainly true of my first hospital antenatal classes, where these various gadgets such as the epidural infuser and amniohook were passed around for all of us fearful mothers to handle in hushed silence. My best friend Lisa, as birth partner, came along with me to heckle the 'teachers' with their flip charts. Even though Lisa had breastfed her own two boys until aged two, she disagreed with the midwives' bullying stance on breast-feeding, a view that caused at least one mother who wanted to bottle-feed never to return.

Less biased than the hospital classes are the NCT class-es, an acronym that stands for *National* Childbirth Trust, not *Natural* Childbirth Trust as many think (so you are not going to be asked to get on all fours and moo like a cow). NCT classes offer mothers the oppor-tunity to meet up after the birth, share their experiences and become friends. This is no small matter when the realization of having to look after your deeply-desired little darling sets in. Parenting always seems less daunt-ing when it is done in a group with coffee and chocolate biscuits around. To join an NCT antenatal group, tele-phone 0870 444 8707.

If you are looking for something a little bit different, why not set up your own group and start sculpting or painting with pregnant women, using the sugges-tions from the *Birthing from Within* book (visit www.birthingfromwithin.com for details of how to hold a workshop). Even antenatal yoga groups or Hyp-nobirthing sessions with other pregnant women, or informal coffee mornings with new mothers and mothers-to-be, can be instructive and reassuring.

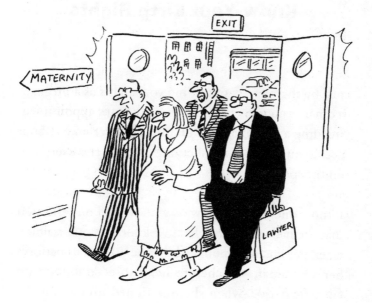

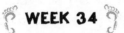

Know Your Birth Rights

Just by the very act of reading your rights as a pregnant woman, you will enter your next doctor's appointment standing a little bit taller. Or, perhaps later on in labour itself, you might remember one of them and exercise it on the spot.

I know one mother of twins who wished on reflection that she had used her rights to ask for a second opinion when her doctor announced that he wanted to perform her Caesarean well before her babies' due date on Christmas Eve (when she questioned him about the necessity, she was told that she was being 'selfish'). It may have suited the doctor to have her case out of the way before he went on his Christmas holidays, but it certainly added to her burden. Now she has to organize two birthdays before the biggest holiday of the year.

Difficult as it may be to believe, we probably have more rights as pregnant women in this country than the women in any other country in the world. You have the right to refuse scans or any type of treatment you don't want – and even to have someone ejected from the room in labour if you don't like the look of them (my friend Sue wished she had known this when she caught a student nurse flirting with her husband while she was contracting away on the bed). Should you really dig your heels in, the law will almost always come out in your favour. When a woman refused to be induced at 36 weeks for suspected pre-eclampsia, the doctor tried to get a court order for a Caesarean by telling the judge it was an emergency. Following the section, the woman appealed and the appeal court ruled the hospital's action was unlawful and awarded her £40,000. Afterwards the High Court issued guidelines for all medical professionals reminding them that a woman has the right to refuse treatment and cannot be forced to undergo it unless they can clearly demonstrate she is not rational.

Having all these rights is wonderful in theory but hopeless in practice if you *hate* to make a fuss or cause embarrassment. If you can't face it, get your partner, husband or someone who likes a bit of confrontation to help your cause. Or remember that making a fuss is getting you in 'embarrassment training' for toddler tantrums at the supermarket checkout.

Current Government policy in the UK means that you are entitled to the following [adapted from the Government's Changing Childbirth manifesto, 1993]:

- To opt for midwifery care only
- To have a home birth
- To refuse to be attended by anyone you do not wish present, such as a medical student (I politely asked a student to wait outside for my second doctor's appointment because I didn't feel I had the doctor's proper attention)
- A second opinion
- A copy of the research paper that supports the advice you are being given
- A copy of the hospital protocol or guidelines for the relevant aspect of your care – e.g. induction of labour (I asked for the Twin Birth protocol from my hospital and was able to clarify what some of the medical jargon meant with my doctor)
- To refuse any treatment that you do not wish to receive (when I asked Beverley Beech, who runs the Association for Improvements in the Maternity Services, how you do this, she suggested bringing along a door wedge to the delivery suite)
- To have a copy of your records and the correspondence about your case (free if you apply within 40 days of your last consultation)

These are your rights, so don't be afraid to use them. If you do, your story might help the next mother who comes after you, and who may be unaware that she has any. Don't be afraid to challenge the hospital's authority if you are unhappy with what you are being told. It is in the hospital's interest, not yours, to have all of us women in labour in a single maternity ward, served by fewer midwives than if we were at home or in a Birth Centre.

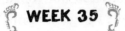

Write Your Birth Plan

Home-made birth plans, rather than the hospital tick-the-box sort, are a useful tool if you are planning a hospital birth. Although it is only a piece of paper that might be best used as a paper airplane after the event, it is a proper document to discuss with your partner and to talk through with your midwife or doctor at the 36-week appointment. Jo Sweeney, an antenatal teacher at the National Childbirth Trust, suggests making a separate appointment to do this if you run out of time, as many do, at that 36-week check-up.

Doctors in particular, with all those exams they have had to pass, react well to pieces of paper and take you more seriously if pressed to comment. And the very fact that you have typed it up proves that you are not someone to be brushed away with a smile and the ubiquitous 'Let's see what happens on the day.'

Even though a copy of the birth plan will be attached to your notes, do bring in a spare on the day and remind midwives looking after you that **you have thought**

through the issues very carefully and would appreciate their support in getting the help suggested. As one mother commented in a recent maternity journal:

I got this worrying feeling that, even if I said beforehand that I didn't want Syntometrine [an injection to deliver the placenta more quickly] or Vitamin K [a routine baby jab for an extremely rare blood-clotting disorder], at a vulnerable moment they might try to persuade me. And I didn't want to have to deal with that. I wanted my opinions to be respected.[1]

Writing a birth plan and asking the midwife or doctor to sign at the bottom to confirm that they have read it will give some assurance that your views have been listened to. Discussing the specific details you have included will winkle out their views, the hospital guidelines, and where support will come from. It might also bring to light some things you haven't yet discussed with your partner, such as whether you want to find out the sex of the baby yourself at the birth, or be told by the midwife.

What a birth plan should not do is lull you into a false sense of security that the birth will go according to plan, or that your views will be listened to on the day. Think of your birth plan as a research tool and don't become too wedded to it. After all, *you* might change your mind on the day as well. 'Be flexible,' says Jo Sweeney at the NCT, 'if you are rigid about what you want and it doesn't work out that way you might feel disappointed after the birth. Do include issues that are really important to you.'

Here is a modified version of a birth plan that I took to my doctor when expecting twins. When he reacted to one of the points by saying 'If I were you, I wouldn't do that,' I reminded him that he would never be me, up the duff with twins. He smiled.

Birth Plan for a Hospital Birth

Dear doctors, paediatricians and midwives who may be attendant at delivery.

Please find below the requests of my husband and I for labour, delivery and the immediate post-partum period at Chelsea & Westminster Hospital. My husband and I are keen for me to have as little medical intervention as possible during labour and delivery in order to bond with and nurse the babies immediately after birth, and to leave the hospital as soon as we are deemed fit to do so.

[If there is any complication or high-risk element to your baby's delivery, you might want to insert how you have read the hospital guidelines – sometimes called protocols – on, say, breech delivery, and that you still hope for the following.]

While we trust your medical judgement and feel confident that you will support our requests as long as they are medically feasible, we would be most grateful if you would raise any points in the plan that you feel are unacceptable or inadmissible at this early stage.

Our requests include those for a 'normal' birth and those for one with complications. Both assume that **labour will not be induced early, and that the baby will be able to go overdue without insistence on the part of the hospital for routine induction**. [Perhaps if you have healthy examples of babies in your family born at 43 weeks – if so, it might be worth inserting a line about it here.]

I plan in the event of a normal birth:

1 To labour in a pool in the hospital at the beginning of active labour [on my twin birth plan the doctor wrote 'if less than 2-3 cm dilated']
2 To be attended by my husband/mother/sister/aunt, or all of them
3 To be attended during labour by midwives only
4 To have no students observing the birth [if, like me, you are a privacy freak. Remember, too, that unnecessary and unknown people can slow down labour and that this is a sacred rite of passage, not a peep show.]
5 To have access to gas and air as the only form of tranquillizer or pain medication [you may want to add pethidine or an epidural here]
6 To take in homoeopathic remedies, TENS machines, and have reflexology/acupuncture/hypnosis practised on me by my birth assistant

7   To have no routine stimulants such as syntocinon, to start or speed up labour

8   To have no rupture of membranes [breaking of the waters] without my consent

9   To have no routine intravenous drip [sometimes this is put in 'just in case' you need anaesthetic, and to give you additional sugar in a long labour] but to eat and drink as I see fit [food works just as well]

10 To have no routine electronic foetal monitoring, but to have a sonicaid hand-held monitor used instead [controversial, this one – the doctor may quote hospital protocols]

11 To be free to walk around during labour – no routine confinement to the bed or labour room [much easier if you have got consent on not being hooked up to monitors and drips]

12 To be taken to the delivery suite [where you have your baby] from the labour ward [where you labour] with an experienced midwife in attendance

13 To have the option to choose delivery positions: to deliver on my side, hands and knees, squatting, standing up – whatever position feels comfortable at the time

14 To hold the baby immediately on delivery. We do not want the baby put into a warmer, have the mucus sucked out [it drains naturally anyway] or to be given to a paediatrician for inspection first. We would also like to attempt to nurse the baby immediately [babies are often amazingly alert after

birth, and equally amazingly willing to root away at
your nipple].

15 If labour takes longer than the usual hospital protocol, to not feel pressurized 'to get on with it' if both
the baby and myself are doing fine. If epidural is
used, to allow the epidural to wear off and/or the
urge to push commence before being expected to
push.

16 To not be subjected to routine episiotomy and to
have the hospital policy on 'tearing' clearly explained

17 To have a physiological third stage of labour without
injections of ergometrine or infusion of syntocinon
or syntometrine without my agreement [in other
words, to deliver the placenta naturally. The placenta,
which many women forget about after the baby
arrives, slithers out in its own time with one easy
'cough' – mine took 12 minutes for two placentas
after the twins. If you are married to Hugh Fearnley-
Whittingstall and are planning on cooking a placenta
stew, now is the moment to insert that you want to
keep it, and to invite your doctor around]

18 To prevent excess blood-loss and complications in
the third stage by allowing the cord of the baby to
cease pulsating before clamping and separation, and
my [husband/partner/etc.] to clamp the cord [now
you are showing off that you have read all the books
and attended the classes, and the doctor will definitely treat you with extra respect]

In the event of complications during labour and delivery:

1 For the obstetrician to meet the above requests if
   medically feasible
2 If I should have to have a Caesarean birth, to have
   my [husband/partner, etc.] present holding my hand

In the event that the baby might have to require care in
the special care unit [twins are often premature]:

1 To be able to hold the baby, if medically feasible, or
   at least touch him/her before he/she goes to the special care baby unit (SCBU).
2 To have the baby receive breast milk that I pump for
   him/her and to nurse as soon as he/she is able

Signed: Emma and Adam Barker

Signed: midwife/doctor (I have read the above and respect
the mother's/parents' views)

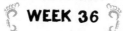

Tour the Hospital

If you are planning to give birth in hospital, a tour of the maternity ward may help allay any fears of the unknown that might spring up on the day. If possible, and the maternity ward allow, try to book a tour that is not with a herd of others and allows you to ask questions as you go along. Ask to see any water pool facilities, and a delivery suite where the birthing might actually take place. Walk to the window, close your eyes and imagine yourself in the room, excited at the prospect of meeting your baby. Ask what you can bring to customize the room, such as aromatherapy oils or music, hypnobirthing tapes or a birth ball, and what the equipment above the bed is for.

If there is anything unusual about your forthcoming birth – say the baby is in breech position or you are carrying twins – ask whether there are any hospital midwives experienced in this type of birth that you might meet. If possible, meet as many of the hospital midwives as you can. They are separate from the community midwives who look after you before and after the birth, although occasionally you may find one of your community midwives on the ward. Try and remember names to personalize the experience as much as possible. The object of the maternity ward tour is to dispel any fears that you may harbour subconsciously about this strange and unfamiliar place. Stay there until your feel comfortable, noting how your body reacts to the place and how you feel.

Glossary of Big Words Doctors Use around Birth

apgar score This is the test performed on newborns immediately after delivery for pinkness and alertness. Scores are given out of 10, and doctors sometimes cite 'lower apgar scores' as a reason to recommend a particular interventionist course of action. Most babies 'pink up nicely' even if their apgar scores are a little low on delivery, however. For example, a recent study on babies born by elective Caesarean and VBAC (vaginal birth after Caesarean) showed that while more VBAC babies had a lower apgar score at 1 minute old (9.6 per cent were under 7, compared to 1.5 per cent of Caesarean babies), the scores were exactly the same at 5 minutes old.

Dilating/Dilation This describes the opening of the cervix in readiness for the baby to come down the birth canal. The measurement used is in centimetres, so you will be described as '2 cm dilated' in very early labour, or '7 cm dilated' when on the way, with the jackpot being '10 cm dilated' – big enough to accommodate a baby's head.

Internal or External Version This is another phrase for the doctor or junior registrar's attempts to 'turn a baby'. So a doctor may manually manipulate the baby externally via the mother's stomach (external version) or by reaching in internally, usually when a woman is anaesthetized in that area.

Stages of Labour

First Stage This is early labour. The contractions may be coming, but in between you are able to walk and talk. Your cervix is opening slowly (or quickly, depending on how your body behaves), and you can still have a bath, eat and move around.

Transition The mini-pause between first and second stage which is sometimes described as the eye of the storm. The transition from first stage to second stage can be quite subtle, but an experienced midwife should be able to recognize it (the transition is sometimes marked by the mother becoming fed up and tired, complaining that 'I can't go on any more!'). However, I know I said this in my labour in the hope that it might mean *I was in transition*.

Second Stage Often quoted as the desire to push, this stage can be relatively short compared to the first stage, and starts when you are fully dilated and the baby is ready to be born.

Third Stage Pushing out the afterbirth – or expelling the placenta, to use the technical term. It seems a bit of a drag that you have yet another job to do after having the baby, but your body will usually do it for you with just a few mini-contractions. Some hospitals insist on giving you an injection of syntometrine to hurry things along – be sure to make it clear whether you want this or not.

Syntocinon A synthetic form of oxytocin, the main hormone that stimulates the uterus to contract. It is given via an intravenous drip and is sometimes used to bring on labour artificially, known as 'induction' or 'inducing' labour. 'We know that induction buggers up women's labours' boomed Caroline Flint, former head of the Royal College of Midwives, on a Radio 4 programme in November 2003, and induction can overstimulate the uterus, starting contractions off that are much stronger and that much more painful to deal with (and therefore triggering the need for more pain-relief or anaesthesia to cope with them), as well as, in rare cases, causing the placenta to come away from the uterine wall. The author Peter Carey, witnessing the effects of syntocinon on his partner in labour, described it as having a 'fast, intense effect, like a double scotch when you're expecting a beer'.

Syntocinon may also be given during labour, if labour is not progressing or contractions are not deemed to be efficient enough (or the hospital just wants to process

you a little more quickly). Finally, it may also be inject-
ed into you after the baby is born to stimulate the
womb to deliver the placenta. If you don't want this to
happen, remember to ask for a 'natural third-stage
delivery of the placenta' on your birth plan, and to
remind the midwife on the day.

Strange Words Midwives Use

Niggling This is when labour is just beginning and the
hormones are up, the mother is a little uncomfortable
and the odd contraction suggests that the baby is on its
way. A midwife might say, 'She's been niggling all day,
but she's not in labour yet.'

Palpating Before the days of scans, midwives used to
'palpate' the mother's stomach to check how the baby
was lying, and whether the head was engaged or the
baby was breech. Even today this is still a good midwifery skill to have.

Pinard/Sonicaid These are less high-tech alternatives
to the slendertone pads of an electronic foetal monitor. Instead of continuous monitoring with a
print-out at the end, hand-held sonicaids allow the
midwife to listen in intermittently to check the baby's
heartbeat. Really old-fashioned sorts might have a
primitive little ear trumpet called a pinard. If you have
a water birth where electric pads can't be used (can't

think why, can you?) then you will be monitored with one of these devices.

To get a bit more technical, pinards enable a practitioner to listen to the actual pumping heart of a baby, while ultrasonic aids (both hand-held and continuous) use the Doppler effect and average out every five beats – the result being that the noise produced sounds a bit like the baby's heartbeat, but isn't.

Poles The baby's head and the bum are at two opposite poles, and this is why the midwife palpates to find out which pole is where.

Rest and Be Thankful This applies to any stage in labour when the contractions 'go off' (another midwives' fave) and things quiet down for no explainable reason. If her observations show that you and the baby are in 'good nick', a midwife might suggest that you Rest and Be Thankful, while a needle-happy doctor might wheel over an IV drip for induction.

Finally, be prepared if your midwife gets you to practise saying things in front of the mirror that you consider outside your comfort zone. My midwife Mary Cronk encourages her clients and any other pregnant women that she comes into contact with to say the following:

1 (To be said with a sweet smile): 'Thank you sooo much for your advice Mr Hi-an-Mitee, we will consider it carefully and let you know OUR decision.'

2 'Perhaps you can let me have the reference to the research paper that supports your opinion.'

3 (To be said with a regretfully less sweet smile): 'I'm afraid I shall have to regard further discussion as harassment.'

4 (To be said firmly): 'Would you like to reconsider what you have just said?' (in response to being told one is a 'silly girl' or 'being a bit selfish' or similar).

5 'STOP THAT AT ONCE!' (in response to any examinations or interventions that you are not yet ready for)

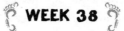

WEEK 38

Women Who Birth Well

If this is your first birth, of course you do not know how labour and birth will progress on the day, but there is still plenty you can do to plan for it. For you the hardest thing will be knowing how your body will react. Here are a few things you can do to make sure that everything goes as smoothly as possible.

- Find out from your mother or sisters how their births went, and what more they might have done to have made them better. We have a peculiar genetic tendency to emulate the birth experiences of our mothers and siblings. My mother told me at a crucial time, after a full day of labour failing to progress with the twins, that she had had exactly the same problem when expecting her twins until the midwife broke her waters. Mid-labour I was able to pass on this information to my midwives, who then offered to break my waters. Once my membranes were ruptured, the twins were born within 40 minutes.
- Try to stay at home as long as possible in the early

part of labour. Generally speaking, the more relaxing your surroundings, the easier it will be for dilation to occur. You should feel a lot more relaxed in your own home, walking around and leaning on the banister when a contraction comes along, than dodging the hospital trolley in the maternity ward corridor. Try to establish before labour starts whether a midwife can visit you at home to examine you in early labour so you don't have to go into the hospital.

- Look forward to it. It may seem weirdly masochistic to say that pain is only a part of birth, but 'pain with a purpose' or 'positive pain', if such phrases exist, are quite different from the stubbing-your-toe sort. We women are better equipped to deal with pain than men, and you will have so many hormones swilling around you on the day that you may be as cool as a cucumber while everyone around you is burning their fingers on the hot water and towels. Enjoy the fuss. A woman in labour is a queen bee. Soon enough you will be elbowed aside for others to get a better view of the baby.

According to the handout from the Common Knowledge Trust (a New Zealand outfit that sells 'The Pink Kit' and can be visited on the Internet at www.commonknowledgetrust.com), all women who birth well do the same things and can explain the following about themselves to others. Remember, all these traits are learned behaviour, not inherited, so there is still time to practise them.

Women who birth well:

1 breathe effectively and in a relaxed manner
2 use their breath to renew themselves with an inhale and to reduce tension with an exhale through nose or mouth
3 use their breath as a focus
4 are aware of how to maintain and recapture relaxation on the inside of their bodies
5 maintain a body posture which facilitates the experience and helps the baby descend through the body
6 are internally aware and can explain what is happening either while in labour or afterwards
7 touch themselves appropriately to facilitate their experience
8 help others to know how to assist them
9 make certain they go into labour rested
10 focus their mental capacity to the task at hand and let other things sit on the side until a more appropriate time
11 focus moment to moment. They do not dwell on the past or future of the experience
12 say 'I know what I am doing' and 'I manage myself well'
13 say 'If I lost it for a moment, I got back on track'

Finally, the Kiwi experts suggest shutting your eyes and repeating the following affirmation: **'To birth well I must give myself fully to the task but I also must let go and let it happen by itself. Women who birth well control their surrender to the process. Birth is learning to control surrender.'**

Repeat after me (preferably while laughing): **'Birth is learning to control surrender.'**

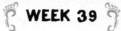

Am I in Labour?

This may seem like a stupid question to ask, but don't be surprised if you find this becomes your mantra as the pregnancy wears on. Somehow we are expected to know whether or not we are in labour, as if a host of angels will suddenly appear to serenade you to the Delivery Suite. The reality is somewhat different. Take the mother who insisted on being driven immediately to the hospital because her seat was wet, thinking her waters had broken in the car, only to find on arrival that she was 'still pregnant' and her husband had mistakenly left open the car window in the rain.

Take also the fact that 'early', 'latent' or even 'false' labour, as it used to be called, can mean that you are still having contractions 5 minutes apart but the contractions are only positioning the baby, or getting the baby's lungs used to the idea of breathing. For this reason, labour is often referred to as 'active' or 'established' when things are really starting to move. But be aware that early labour can involve tightenings which feel like contractions SEVERAL DAYS before you are actually in labour. You feel excited and don't rest well (birth hormones are adrenalin-based and become more active) and are absolutely certain that you are in labour (whether you've had a baby or not). However, **one thing is for certain, you will not be in labour unless the whole business is progressing**. Labour is about progress, the inexorable movement towards the ultimate goal – the body producing a baby. Anything that 'goes off' or 'quiets down' is just limbering up.

This is worth knowing because, if you didn't, you might just wear yourself out before your help is finally needed (pushing, my dear). **What you should be doing is eating well, drinking lots of fluid and resting, resting, resting**. What you are probably doing is running all over the house saying, 'I know I put my maternity pants somewhere, why isn't anybody helping?'

If you can bear it, and the midwives agree, stay at home for as long as possible. Go for little walks, have lovely baths, ask a friend to come over and make you peanut butter and marmite sandwiches, but try not to whizz into hospital on the first contraction. Labour progresses much better when you are relaxed and in your own environment, not hooked up to monitors like the bride of Frankenstein.

Finally, when in active labour at home, keep asking yourself, as if it's your birthday, 'What do I want to do now?' – and then do it.

Physical Signs of Early Labour

Waters breaking: this can either be a small trickle coming from a tear in the amniotic sac or a sudden gush (one mother describes bending down for a tin of baked beans in the supermarket, followed by 'splashdown!') Remember, however, that your waters might not break (officially known as 'rupture of membranes') until you are in established labour, and occasionally babies are born in their amniotic sac (in former times a child 'born in the caul' was believed to be very lucky). When your waters do break, you should tell your midwife immediately. Some hospitals have protocols suggesting you go in straight away, others are happy to let you stay at home, and most will want the baby delivered within the next 72 hours to prevent infection.

Contractions that come 10 or fewer minutes apart, have been going on for at least an hour, and are getting stronger or more frequent. As my midwife Mary Cronk says, 'If you have contractions that come oftener, last longer, get stronger and progress to a state where they are coming too b***dy often, lasting too b***dy long, and are too b***dy strong, then take strength: your baby is nearly here.'

Mucus plug: a glob of period-like stuff that looks just like it sounds. The plug can appear some days before labour starts because the cervix has begun to open and thin out.

Possible Physical Signs of Early Labour

- nagging or intermittent backache
- diarrhoea
- feeling nauseous or flu-like
- increased vaginal discharge
- nesting instinct – the sudden desire to clean the top of the wardrobe or sort out your pants drawer (not reliable indicator for tidy freaks)

What They Don't Tell You to Pack for the Hospital (But What You Really Need)

FOR LABOUR

- Snacks – Suzannah Olivier, author of *Eating for a Perfect Pregnancy* recommends Isotonic sports drinks and glucose drinks to keep your liquid and salt levels up in labour, with soups and juices rather than heavy snacks, so as not to put stress on the digestive tract. I, however, preferred honey sandwiches. Note that the hospital may advise you not to eat if there is a possibility of your needing anaesthetic.

- Bendy straws – in order to drink the glucose drinks at funny angles (like on your hands and knees)
- Slippers (to buff up those greasy NHS floors)
- Your own pillowcase, smelling of your own washing powder, associated with all things pleasant and relaxing
- Disinfectant baby wipes (to wipe loo seats and baths out before you get in)
- *Hello!* or *OK!* magazine – anything more challenging than picture captions to read will be tossed in the bin. Also, these two always have joyous photos of celebs with newborns to ponder alternative baby names ('Maybe Persephone is the new Chloe?')
- Birth ball/calming music tapes/Yellow Homoeopathic Childbirth kit (see page 72/aromatherapy and massage oils/TENS machine/favourite scented candle to keep the air smelling sweet.

FOR AFTER THE BIRTH

- Camera with fast film (for those minutes-after-the baby-is-born snaps)
- New nightie to change into the minute before those minutes-after-the-baby-is-born-snaps
- New dressing-gown for ditto (you don't want to wander the hospital grounds in some embarrassing frayed favourite)

- Pashmina shawls – new fake ones are better than old originals, to wrap up the baby bundle in something other than NHS cellular specials

FOR AN AT-HOME BIRTH

This is the list that I drew up with my midwife for the technical extras for the birth.

- Something waterproof for the floor or bed or sofa or wherever you want to be
- Old sheeting if available, or old towels
- A roll of cotton wool.
- A box of man-sized tissues
- Pudding basin or similar to fit inside your largest saucepan
- Nourishing snacks
- Nourishing drinks of choice
- Nice music of choice
- Camera with fast film
- Labour nightie
- Favourite scented candle
- Packet of disposable nappies
- Maternity pads and pants
- Bin liners
- Bucket

(The midwife brings a small blue bag containing the pethidine, and something resembling a diver's tank has the gas and air.)

So, your bag is packed, your house is clean, the nursery has an empty Moses basket awaiting the new arrival, now all that's left is for me to wish you luck and say goodbye. If you've read this far, you're well prepared for what's ahead, even if you secretly still feel you're settling in for a night of *Scary Movie 2*.

Somebody's words, somewhere in the book will come back to you when you most need them. Giving birth is a joyous rite of passage, and henceforth you will connect with other women in a way that you have never done so before. You are a lucky, lucky person – so lucky that I wish I could do it for you. But I can't. It's something that you have to do for yourself, and you will come out the other side a woman, no longer a girl. Birth is your introduction to motherhood, the sweat and the tears to follow, and no-one should take it away from you. So I send you on your way with all the love in the world for you and your soon-to-be-born baby. Thanks for listening. God Bless.

References

First Stage – Let's Start at the Very Beginning …

A VERY GOOD PLACE TO START …

1   Ina May Gaskin, *Ina May's Guide to Childbirth* (Random House, 2003)
2   Peter Brocklehurst, director of the National Perinatal Epidemiology Unit, in the *Independent* 22 October 2003

LET'S TALK ABOUT SEX, BABY

1   *Birthing Your Baby, The Second Stage* (AIMS publication, March 2001): page 30

MY BODY IS A TEMPLE

1   Sarah Blaffer Hardy, 'An infant's eye view', in *Mother Nature: Maternal instincts and how they shape the human species* (Vintage, 2000): page 434
2   Suzannah Olivier, *Eating for a Perfect Pregnancy* (Simon & Schuster Pocket Books, 2001)
3   G. Nowak and B. Szewczyk, 'Mechanisms contributing to antidepressant zinc actions'; S. R. De Vriese, A. B. Christophe

and M Maes, 'Lowered serum n-3 polyunsaturated fatty acid (PUFA) levels predict the occurrence of postpartum depression' (www.ncbi.nlm.nih.gov:80/entrez)

4   Denise Tiran, *Natural Remedies for Morning Sickness and Other Pregnancy Problems* (Quadrille Press, 2001): page 159

5. 'Aromatherapy Pregnancy', *The Professional* November 2003 – Debbie Hilder, an aromatherapist from Truro, performed her case-study on 39-year-old pregnant woman in the last fours weeks of pregnancy

6   Denise Tiran, *Natural Remedies for Morning Sickness and Other Pregnancy Problems* (Quadrille Press, 2001): page 30

CAN YOU FEEL IT?

1   Marshall and Phyllis Klaus and John Kennell, *Mothering the Mother* (Da Capo Press, 1993)

2   Marshall and Phyllis Klaus and John Kennell, *Mothering the Mother* (Da Capo Press, 1993): page 45

3   Beverley Beech, reported in *Midwifery Digest* December 2000: pages 467– 9

4   Marshall H. Klaus and John H. Kennell, *Maternal-Infant Bonding: The Impact of Early Separation or Loss on Family Development* (St Louis: C. V. Mosby Co., 1976)

5   Marshall and Phyllis Klaus and John Kennell, *Mothering the Mother* (Da Capo Press, 1993): page 44

6   Marshall and Phyllis Klaus and John Kennell, *Mothering the Mother* (Da Capo Press, 1993): page 112

AWAY WITH THE FAIRIES

1   *AIMS Journal,* vol 10, no.2, 1998.

Second Stage - Birth Stories: Brilliant Ways to Give Birth

INTRODUCTION: WATER, WATER EVERYWHERE

1   Michel Odent, 'Birth Under Water', *The Lancet*, 24–31 December, 1983, pages: 1476-7
2   'Water births better for mothers and babies, study shows', the *Independent*, 26 January 2004

CAESAREAN BIRTH

1   Kate Figes, *Life After Birth* (Penguin, 2000)
2   *AIMS Journal*, vol. 16, no.3, 2004: page 12

Third Stage - Eight Weeks to Go

WEEK 35: WRITE YOUR BIRTH PLAN

1   *AIMS Journal*, vol. 15, no. 3, 2003: page 11

Recommended Reading

Before the Birth

(After the baby arrives, reading the front of a newspaper will be a major achievement.)

BOOKS FROM ACROSS THE POND

Spiritual Midwifery (Book Publishing Company, 2002). First published in the 1970s, this book documents an idealistic 1960s' birth culture that proved that support and kindness can produce some of the best birth outcomes recorded anywhere in the developed world. A quirky classic.

Ina May's Guide to Childbirth (Random House, 2003). As a long-awaited sequel to *Spiritual Midwifery*, Ina May offers plenty of the right information to reassure the ordinary primagravida that her 'body is not a lemon'.

Birthing from Within by Pam England and Rob Horowitz (Partera Press, 1998). A rare and original approach to birth that includes stories from a workshop in New Mexico where singing, dancing, drawing and drumming are the norm. A breath of fresh air after an average NCT class.

Best Friend's Guide to Pregnancy: Or Everything Your Doctor Won't Tell You by Vicki Iovine (Bloomsbury, 1997). Vicki Iovine deserves the American equivalent of an OBE for services to womankind for writing this lighthearted guide to pregnancy. The only sadness is that she was wheeled in for a Caesarean, so whizzes over birth rather quickly.

Mothering the Mother: How a Doula Can Help You Have a Shorter, Easier and Healthier Birth by Marshall H. Klaus et al, (Da Capo Press, 1993). Get this if you are considering it.

HOME-GROWN MANUALS

From Here to Maternity by Mel Giedroyc (Ebury Press, 2004) At last, a British Vicki Iovine who offers a personal, extremely funny romp through her first pregnancy from beginning to normal birth at the end. I defy you not to laugh.

Becoming a Mother: an essential guide to the facts, feelings and emotions of pregnancy and birth by Kate Mosse (Virago, 1993). A sensitive and searching discussion on the good and bad bits of pregnancy, dealing particularly well with emotional issues that arise as birth approaches.

Birth Your Way: choosing birth at home or in a birth centre by Sheila Kitzinger (Dorling Kindersley, 2002). Useful reading if you are thinking of doing either of the above, and mercifully free of the graphic photographs of beardy weirdies that usually pepper DK's birth books.

New Pregnancy and Birth Book by Dr Miriam Stoppard (Ballantine Books, 2000). If you need a comprehensive guide to please the mother-in-law, this is one of the best to get, although the 1970s' photos are a no-no for me, and the diagrams send me into an O level Biology revision crisis.

Preparing for Birth with Yoga by Janet Balaskas (HarperCollins, 2003). Simple exercises for an Active Birth from the woman who has spent 25 years practising what she preaches.

AIMS booklets: Ultrasound? Unsound; Am I Allowed?; Induction: Do I Really Need It?; Birth After Caesarean (all available from the Aims Publication Secretary, Manor Barn, Thurloxton, Taunton, Somerset TA2 8RH). For specific aspects of maternity care and for independent advice without any political bias, the volunteer-run Association for Improvement in Maternity Services have the best pamphlets around. They cost a few pounds, and for the full list, apply above or visit www.aims.org.uk

To Save Until after the Birth

A Life's Work: on becoming a mother by Rachel Cusk (Fourth Estate, 2002). Wonderfully written and painfully witty memoir that makes your bath water run cold as you read on and on and on.

A Better Woman by Susan Johnson (Simon & Schuster, 2002) Beautiful and lyrical response to motherhood that is honest, harrowing and utterly absorbing.

How Not to Be A Perfect Mother by Libby Purves (Thorsons, 2004). Nearly twenty years old, but still as fresh as the day it was written, this right rollicking read will knock you flat with its good sense and wise words. A must if returning to work.

All are available from www.amazon.co.uk